Overcoming
Urinary
Incontinence

A Woman's Guide
to Treatment

Michael H. Safir, M.D. ~ Clay N. Boyd, M.D.
Tony E. Pinson, M.D.

Addicus Books
Omaha, Nebraska

An Addicus Nonfiction Book

ISBN 978-1-886039-87-2
Cover design by Peri Poloni Gabriel
Illustrations by Jack Kusler
Typography by Linda Dageforde

This book is not intended to serve as a substitute for a physician. Nor is it the authors' intent to give medical advice contrary to that of an attending physician.

Library of Congress Cataloging-in-Publication Data
Safir, Michael H., 1967-
    Overcoming urinary incontinence : a woman's guide to treatment / Michael H. Safir, Clay N. Boyd, Tony E. Pinson.
        p. cm.
Includes index.
ISBN-13: 978-1-886039-87-2 (alk. paper)
1. Urinary incontinence—Treatment—Popular works. 2. Women—Diseases—Treatment—Popular works. I. Boyd, Clay N., 1961- II. Pinson, Tony E., 1961- III. Title.
    RC921.I5S34 2008
    616.6'2—dc22

                                                    2007036266

Addicus Books, Inc.
P.O. Box 45327
Omaha, Nebraska 68145
www.AddicusBooks.com
Printed in the United States of America
10 9 8 7 6 5 4 3 2 1

Contents

Acknowledgments

My two most important roles are as husband to my wife, Robyn, and father to my children, Julia and Jack. I am the physician I have become because of their sacrifice and support. I honor my mentors, Shlomo Raz, M.D., Jack W. McAninch, M.D., and Anthony Schaeffer, M.D. This book is, in large part, the product of Frances Sharpe who has served as editor and who now knows more about incontinence than any layperson should.

—Michael H. Safir, M.D.

I would like to acknowledge my wife, Dr. Bonnie Accardo Boyd, who has helped weather the storms both pre- and post-Katrina. I also want to thank Dr. Jack C. Winters for all of his energy and expertise, Dr. Richard Airhart for his integrity and determination throughout the storms, Dr. Rodney Appel for his practical role as a dynamic educator, Dr. Joseph Aloysius LaNasa, who has been both friend and mentor, and finally the patients, families, and medical staff throughout the River Parishes for their faith and commitment in rebuilding and supporting the recovering communities.

—Clay N. Boyd, M.D.

I would like to thank my wife Lorna and my children Evan and Alec for their devotion, patience, and support of my professional and personal endeavors, which have often required sacrifice on their parts. Thank you to Cathy Kulpinski and the staff members of Pinson Urology and Continence Center for their tireless work in caring for our patients. I also wish to acknowledge the exceptional staff members of W.A. Foote Memorial Hospital, especially Judy Gillman and Nancy Wilkins. I am also indebted to my patients who inspire me on a daily basis. Finally I would like to thank Frances Sharpe for her editorial assistance in bringing this book to life.

—Tony E. Pinson, M.D.

Introduction

Millions of women have urinary incontinence, but they rarely talk about it. That's because the involuntary loss of urine can be so embarrassing that many women are too ashamed to discuss it—even with a doctor. This means that millions of women, and perhaps you as well, are suffering in silence from a condition that is treatable and, in some instances, curable. In fact, as many as 90 percent of women with incontinence avoid seeking medical help for the problem. Instead, you may alter your daily life, shying away from social occasions or stopping physical exercise for fear of wetting yourself. But you don't need to live your life this way. By seeking help and starting treatment, you may be able to return to your normal activities and enhance your quality of life.

The purpose of this book is to provide you with an easy-to-understand overview of incontinence and its causes, to encourage you to seek help from a medical professional, and to offer information on the numerous treatment options available. We hope this book will inspire you to stop accepting incontinence as a fact of life and start finding a treatment plan that works for you.

Part I

Incontinence: An Overview

Chapter 1

Understanding Incontinence

A re you frustrated because you can't always control when you urinate? When you cough or sneeze, are you worried that urine might leak out? When you feel the urge to urinate, are you afraid you won't make it to the bathroom in time? If so, you aren't alone. Urinary incontinence is a common problem for millions of women. However, like many of these women, you may be too embarrassed to talk about it or even admit that you have a problem. In fact, you may feel that incontinence is something you just have to deal with. *But it isn't!* The more you understand about incontinence, the more you'll realize that it isn't considered normal and it isn't something you have to tolerate.

Incontinence is simply the involuntary loss of urine. The amount of urine that leaks out and the frequency with which leakage occurs can vary greatly from woman to woman. You may dribble a few drops of urine, or you may experience uncontrollable wetting. You may experience leakage only occasionally, or you may find that it's become an everyday occurrence. No matter where you fall in this spectrum, the loss of urine is a problem that should be addressed.

The Female Urinary System

The urinary system processes your body's liquid waste by creating, storing, and eliminating urine. The system consists of the kidneys, the *ureters*, the bladder, the urethra, the *urethral sphincter*, and the pelvic floor muscles.

When the system is working normally, the kidneys filter the body's liquids to create urine. The urine flows from the kidneys through two tubes called ureters that connect the kidneys to the bladder. The bladder stores the urine until you are ready to urinate. The urethral sphincter muscle is normally closed tightly to keep urine in the bladder until you are ready to urinate. The urethra is a short tube that carries the urine out of the body.

When you urinate, muscles in the bladder contract or tighten, forcing the urine out of the bladder. At the same time, the urethral sphincter and the pelvic floor muscles relax, causing the urethra to open to allow urine to flow through it. When your urinary system is working properly, you can delay urination when a bathroom isn't nearby. When you feel the urge to urinate but can't get to the bathroom, your pelvic floor muscles tighten to keep the urethra closed.

Normal urination also involves the nervous system. When your bladder is almost full, sacral nerves send a signal to your brain to alert you that it is time to urinate. Typically, the nerves send a signal before the bladder is completely full, giving you time to get to the bathroom while the bladder continues to fill.

Types of Urinary Incontinence

You may be surprised to discover that there are five types of urinary incontinence. Leakage is a symptom that is associated with all types of urinary incontinence. However, the things that trigger the leakage and the kind of leakage you experience (a few drops, a constant dribble, or the complete emptying of your bladder) depend on which type of incontinence you have. In some cases, you may experience more than one type of incontinence. The five different types of incontinence are: stress incontinence, urge incontinence/overactive bladder, overflow incontinence, functional incontinence, and mixed incontinence.

Female Urinary System

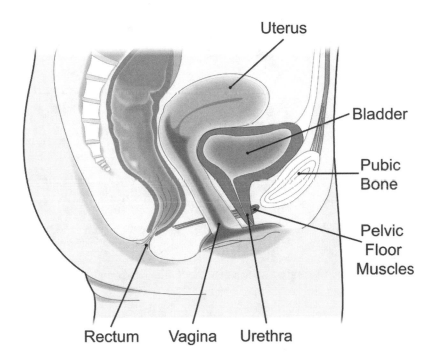

Uterus

Bladder

Pubic Bone

Pelvic Floor Muscles

Rectum   Vagina   Urethra

Stress Incontinence

If you have stress incontinence, you may leak urine when you cough, sneeze, laugh, exercise, get up from sitting, or lift something heavy. The most common type of incontinence women experience, stress incontinence doesn't have anything to do with emotional stress. Its name comes from the fact that these activities put increased intra-abdominal pressure—or stress—on the bladder and the urethra. When you cough or sneeze, it's as if someone were squeezing your bladder from the inside. If the urethra doesn't close tightly enough to keep urine in the bladder when these pressures occur, urine leaks out.

Stress Incontinence

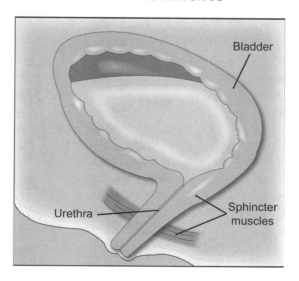

This illustration shows the bladder neck closing normally. No urine is leaking.

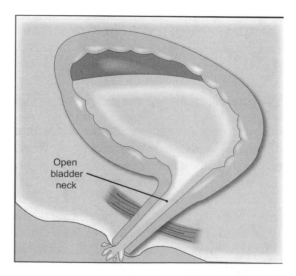

With stress incontinence, the sphincter muscles have weakened, allowing urine to leak.

Urge Incontinence and Overactive Bladder

If you feel sudden, overwhelming urges to urinate, you may have urge incontinence. With urge incontinence, the feeling that you need to urinate comes on so suddenly, you may have only a matter of seconds before your bladder empties uncontrollably. Unfortunately, you simply don't always have enough time to get to the bathroom before an accident occurs.

Urge incontinence may be triggered when you get up from a chair or when you drink even a small amount of liquid. It can also be triggered by what is referred to as the "key-in-the-lock" syndrome. This occurs when you experience an overwhelming urge to urinate when you start to open the door upon arriving home. It's the anticipation of being able to relieve yourself once you arrive home that brings on the uncontrollable urge the second you put that key in the lock. In some instances, the simple act of putting your hands under running water or even just hearing running water may spark the urge to urinate.

If you feel the urge to urinate frequently, perhaps even as often as once every hour during the day, this is called overactive bladder or urinary frequency. With overactive bladder, you feel the need to urinate even though your bladder isn't full. In fact, you may only eliminate small amounts of urine with each trip to the bathroom. With overactive bladder, you may also wake up several times a night feeling like you have to go. This is called *nocturia.*

Overflow Incontinence

If you drip urine constantly, you may have overflow incontinence. With overflow incontinence, your bladder never completely empties. This leads to an accumulation of urine in the bladder. When the amount of urine exceeds the bladder's capacity, the extra urine—the overflow—pushes the urethra open and leaks out. With overflow incontinence, you may feel like you need to empty your bladder but can't, or you may feel like you never fully empty your bladder when you urinate. You may find that when you try to empty your bladder, you have trouble starting or the stream of urine is weak. Overflow incontinence is the least common type of incontinence among women.

Functional Incontinence

If you have normal control over your bladder but you have trouble getting to the bathroom in time or getting your clothes off in time, you may have what's known as functional incontinence. For instance, if you're elderly and the bathroom is upstairs, you may not be able to climb the stairs fast enough to prevent an accident. If you have arthritis, you may not be able to unfasten your pants or skirt quickly enough to avoid leakage. In addition, severe mental conditions, such as Alzheimer's disease, can limit the ability to react to the urge to urinate, resulting in functional incontinence.

Mixed Incontinence

When you experience more than one type of incontinence, it's called mixed incontinence. Mixed incontinence is fairly common among women and in most cases, involves a combination of stress and urge incontinence. In some instances, you may begin experiencing both types of incontinence at the same time. In other cases, you may develop one type first and then develop the other type later. It's common for one type to cause stronger symptoms than the other.

Common Questions about Incontinence

■ Who is at risk for becoming incontinent?

Most women think that urinary incontinence is something that only older adults experience, but any woman can become incontinent. It can affect you whether you're young, middle-aged, or in your golden years. Incontinence doesn't discriminate. Women of all ethnicities and in every part of the world are at risk for developing this common condition. Likewise, you can be at risk regardless of your economic status, your education level, or your level of physical fitness.

■ How common is incontinence in women?

Researchers have had a difficult time pinpointing exact numbers, but most experts agree that at least 10 million women in the United States have incontinence. Why has it been so hard to get concrete numbers? Mainly because women are so ashamed and embarrassed about the condition that they're reluctant to talk about it. Because of this, the statistics currently available are all over the map. For instance, the National Institutes of Health reports that 50 percent of all women have occasional bouts of leakage, and that about 20 percent of women over the age of seventy-five experience leakage on a daily basis. The National Kidney and Urologic Diseases Information Clearinghouse estimates that 38 percent of women over the age of sixty have incontinence. Another study indicates that 10 to 30 percent of women ages fifteen to sixty-four are affected by the condition. Still another study shows that one in four women over the age of eighteen experience the involuntary leakage of urine.

Even though estimates vary, experts agree that incontinence is far more common in women than in men. Studies report that women suffer from the condition at twice the rate as men. And no matter how many women are estimated to have incontinence, the numbers are probably higher because so many women are either too embarrassed to admit they have a problem with leakage or simply don't recognize that they have a problem.

■ How many times a day does a woman normally urinate?

Over a twenty-four-hour period, you should urinate an average of five to eight times, approximately once every two to five hours. Each time you go, the stream of urine should last at least ten seconds. For most women, that amounts to about ten

9

to fifteen ounces of urine. The average bladder can hold about twenty ounces of urine.

Certain things can cause you to urinate more frequently throughout the day. For instance, caffeinated beverages, alcohol, and certain medications can increase urine production, causing you to urinate more often. In addition, if you drink large amounts of water or other beverages, you'll likely need to urinate more often. In today's society, the accepted rule of thumb is to drink at least eight eight-ounce glasses of water a day and to drink *before* you feel thirsty. But these trendy notions are flawed. So how much should you drink each day? Expert opinions vary but you should aim for about four to eight eight-ounce glasses of fluid per day, and you should let thirst be your guide. Don't forget that fluids, such as the milk you put in your cereal and the broth in soups, can count toward your overall daily fluid intake.

■ Is needing to urinate several times during the night considered normal?

Waking up once or twice at the most with the urge to urinate is a common occurrence and is considered normal. If you have to get up more than twice a night to urinate, you may have a problem. If you drink a lot of liquids in the evening, you're more likely to feel the urge to urinate at night. If this is the case, you may want to drink most of your liquids during the morning and afternoon and limit your fluid intake in the evening.

■ Is it normal to have to push or strain to empty the bladder?

There should be no need to push or strain to empty the bladder. The stream should flow comfortably. In fact, urination shouldn't be something you have to think about. If your body is functioning normally, you typically won't even be aware of the number of times you go to the bathroom to urinate, and the mechanics involved in urination probably won't be something you think about. However, if you're conscious of how often you're going or you've noticed anything about the mechanics (pushing, straining, starting and stopping, dribbling, difficulty getting the flow started), you may have a problem.

■ Does incontinence come on suddenly, or does it occur gradually?

Stress and urge incontinence tend to develop gradually and worsen over time. At first, you may leak only a few drops of urine on rare occasions. As time passes, however, you may discover that you're leaking greater amounts on a more frequent basis. Or you may initially experience urinary frequency, which makes you feel like you have to urinate more than normal, but no leakage. This can progress to urge incontinence, where your urge to urinate sometimes results in leakage. Although this gradual pattern is typical, incontinence can also occur suddenly. For example, temporary incontinence is more likely to occur suddenly.

■ Is incontinence a temporary problem or is it a permanent condition?

In some cases, incontinence is a temporary problem. In other instances, it is a long-term condition. Temporary incontinence, which is also called *transient incontinence*, is typically treatable. *Persistent incontinence*, which is also called established incontinence, usually doesn't go away on its own. Whether the incontinence you're experiencing is temporary or persistent depends on the underlying causes.

■ Is incontinence a normal part of aging?

Many women think that urinary incontinence is a normal part of aging, but it isn't. In fact, most women over the age of sixty do not have incontinence. In most cases, incontinence can be prevented or treated, meaning you don't have to live with the fear of leakage. Even so, many women feel resigned that incontinence is a fact of life and simply tolerate it when it

11

occurs. Instead of giving in to incontinence, speak to your family doctor, primary care physician, or gynecologist to gain an understanding of what is and isn't normal. If needed, one of these physicians can refer you to an incontinence specialist.

■ Does incontinence lead to other physical problems?

Leakage and sudden urges to urinate may pose additional physical problems. For instance, lingering wetness can cause a urinary tract infection or skin rashes. In addition, if you're older, you may be more at risk for a fall if you're trying to rush to the bathroom when you feel a sudden urge to urinate.

■ How does incontinence affect overall quality of life?

Considering that incontinence can affect your psychological well-being, your social life, your sex life, and even your career choices, it's no surprise that it can have a tremendous impact on your overall quality of life. In fact, according to studies about how certain diseases and conditions affect your quality of life, incontinence ranks as one of the most devastating.

■ Is one's work life affected by incontinence?

Incontinence can affect every aspect of your life, even your career. Having to urinate frequently or rush to the bathroom when you feel a sudden urge or when you have an accident can be disruptive to your job. In addition, incontinence may play a role in your career choices. For instance, you may pass up promotions or new job opportunities that would require you to travel. Or you may choose a job based on the fact that you'll have easy access to a bathroom. These concerns can prevent you from being successful at and getting ahead in your career.

■ How does incontinence affect one's social life?

The inability to control your bladder can have a negative impact on your social life. If you're like many women with incontinence, you may avoid social situations because you're afraid you'll leak. You may find yourself mapping out your day's activities according to where you can find public bathrooms. You may have to tote around pads or a change of clothes in case of an accident. You may no longer want to go to events where you might have to wait in line to use the restroom. You may stop exercising or you might even try to refrain from laughing in an effort to avoid leakage. You may start avoiding any trips that take you away from the house for more than a short period of time. If you're on the dating scene, the fear of leakage can greatly inhibit your willingness to go out on dates or meet new people. This kind of social withdrawal can dramatically affect your relationships with friends and family.

■ What is the effect of incontinence on one's sex life?

Unexpected leaking during intercourse can be a traumatic experience. Likewise, feeling the urge to urinate during intercourse can put a damper on sexual intimacy. If you leak during sexual relations, or even if you're just afraid that you might leak, you may choose to avoid intimacy with your partner.

■ Is it possible for incontinence to affect one's mental health?

Leakage or simply the fear of wetting yourself can take a devastating emotional toll. In fact, the shame and embarrassment associated with incontinence can be overwhelming and may lead to low self-esteem, anxiety, or even depression. The longer you live with incontinence without seeking help, the more likely you are to have these feelings. Incontinence can make you feel helpless, incapable of controlling your bladder.

■ **Is there help available to treat incontinence?**

The good news is that you can find help for controlling incontinence. Start by recognizing that leakage is a problem, admitting that you have this problem, and seeking treatment for it.

Chapter 2

Causes of Incontinence

Y ou may be surprised to discover that there are a wide variety of reasons why you may be suffering from incontinence. Most medical experts break down incontinence into two categories: *temporary* and *persistent*. Temporary incontinence can often be reversed with treatment and sometimes with nothing more than lifestyle changes. Persistent incontinence, on the other hand, is a long-term problem that is likely to get worse unless treated. Pinpointing what is contributing to your symptoms is an important step in finding a solution to the problem.

Causes of Persistent Incontinence

Common causes of persistent incontinence include poor structural support of the pelvic organs, aging, menopause, hysterectomy and other pelvic surgeries, *pelvic organ prolapse*, urinary tract obstruction, genetic factors, neurological conditions, spinal injuries, nerve damage following radiation, and urinary tract abnormalities. In most cases of persistent incontinence, your symptoms can be dramatically improved with treatment even if the underlying cause persists.

Poor Structural Support of the Pelvic Organs

Proper bladder function relies on healthy functioning of the pelvic muscles and adequate support of the pelvic organs. Damage to the support and function of pelvic muscles is one of the most common causes of urinary incontinence.

For example, the muscles of the pelvic floor must be strong enough to contract sufficiently in order to allow you to hold your urine when you feel the urge to urinate but aren't near a bathroom. If your muscles have been weakened or damaged, they may not be able to contract adequately. In addition, damaged or weakened muscles that do not offer sufficient support to specific areas of the bladder and urethra may lead to stress incontinence.

Having weakened or damaged pelvic muscles has nothing to do with your level of physical fitness. In fact, even if you are in top physical condition, you can still have a weak pelvic floor. Conversely, being less physically fit does not mean that you are more likely to have weakened or damaged pelvic muscles. Several conditions that can damage or weaken the muscles of the pelvic floor include the following:

- Pelvic surgery (such as a hysterectomy)
- Pregnancy and childbirth
- Hormonal deficit
- General injury
- Injury to specific pelvic nerves
- Bed rest
- Pelvic fracture

Aging

The simple act of aging does not necessarily cause incontinence. However, the effects of aging may increase your chances of developing symptoms of urgency, frequency, or leakage of urine. Health problems, such as arthritis, are more common in the elderly and can prevent you from reaching the bathroom in time or getting your clothes off before you have an accident. In some instances, your bladder may lose some of its ability to store urine, or the amount of urine your bladder can store may decrease.

Menopause

Going through menopause or having a hysterectomy may increase your chances of developing incontinence. Postmenopausal women experience decreased production of estrogen, a hormone that's key to maintaining the health of the tissues of the pelvic floor. The reduction in estrogen may cause a thinning in the tissues of the vagina, urethra, and bladder.

In some instances, the damaged tissues are no longer able to close completely, raising the risk of leakage. Thinning of the urethral tissues is associated with a "stiffening" of the urethra, meaning it loses its ability to contract and expand as needed for normal urination. This contributes to symptoms of urge incontinence. The thinning tissues may also cause bladder irritation, which can cause urgency.

Hysterectomy and Pelvic Surgeries

In some cases, having a hysterectomy can raise your risk of developing incontinence. Hysterectomy is one of the most common surgical procedures performed in the United States, and about 40 percent of women over the age of sixty have had the operation. Hysterectomy can affect your bladder control in a number of ways. For instance, a hysterectomy alters the support of the pelvis, leading to a weakness of ligaments that are crucial for preventing incontinence.

Depending on the type of hysterectomy you have had, you may experience a decrease in estrogen production following your surgery. This can occur regardless of your age and is typically associated with hysterectomies that involve the removal of the ovaries in addition to the uterus. The decrease in estrogen produces the same thinning of the tissues of the pelvic floor that can occur in postmenopausal women.

Hysterectomies performed due to uterine or ovarian cancer pose additional risks. For example, they increase the risk of damaging the sacral nerves that allow the bladder to signal the urge to urinate. If you aren't feeling the urge to urinate even though your bladder is full, you're more likely to experience leakage.

Causes of Incontinence

Urge Incontinence

- Bladder irritants (foods and beverages)
- Nerve damage
- Bladder infection
- Cystitis
- Bladder stones
- Bladder tumors
- Medications
- Stool impaction
- Dehydration
- Urinary retention
- Delirium
- Large fluid intake
- Smoking
- Excessive bathroom breaks
- Cold temperatures

Mixed Incontinence

- Combination of causes

Overflow Incontinence

- Nerve damage
- Medications
- Stool impaction
- Obstruction (rare in women)
- Diabetes

Functional Incontinence

- Restricted mobility

Stress Incontinence

- Pregnancy and childbirth
- Hormonal deficit
- Previous pelvic surgery
- Pelvic organ prolapse
- Urinary retention
- High-impact exercise
- Lack of physical exercise
- Being overweight or obese
- Nerve root compression

If you already had incontinence prior to having a hysterectomy, your symptoms may improve, worsen, or remain the same following the procedure. Studies on postoperative symptoms in women who were already incontinent show that a hysterectomy can have unpredictable results.

Any surgery in the pelvic area can affect the muscles of the pelvic floor or the nerves of the urinary system and, subsequently, your ability to control your bladder. Pelvic operations can also result in adhesions and scarring to the exterior of the bladder, which can affect urinary control. In general, the more extensive the operation you've had, the higher your risk for postoperative incontinence. Pelvic operations other than hysterectomy include procedures involving the colon and reconstruction of pelvic fractures. In some instances, postoperative incontinence is only temporary and improves with time. In other cases, it becomes a chronic problem.

Pelvic Organ Prolapse

Pelvic organ prolapse occurs when one or more of the organs within the pelvis drops out of its normal position and bulges or protrudes into the vaginal wall. The bladder is the most common organ to prolapse, but other organs, such as the

Cystocle

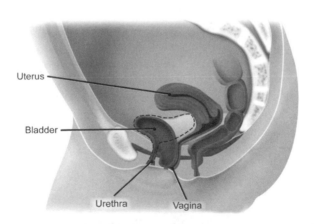

©ETHICON, INC. Reproduced with permission

The most common type of pelvic organ prolapse, a prolapsed bladder, is called a cystocele. It occurs when the wall between the bladder and the vagina weakens, allowing the bladder to droop into the vagina. Above, the dotted line indicates where the normal bladder lies.

19

Uterine Prolapse

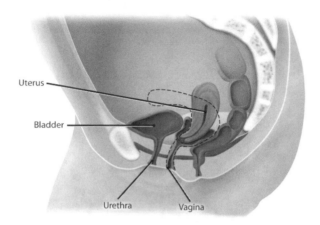

Uterus

Bladder

Urethra   Vagina

A uterine prolapse occurs when the uterus drops from its normal position within the pelvis into the vagina. The dotted line shows where the uterus normally lies.

uterus or rectum, can prolapse as well. The most common causes of prolapse include pregnancy, childbirth, menopause, aging, genetics, obesity, and previous surgery.

Pelvic organ prolapse is common among women, with an estimated 34 million women affected by the condition. Approximately 11 percent of all women will have surgery to correct the condition prior to the age of eighty. Pelvic organ prolapse often results in urinary problems, such as an interrupted or slow urinary stream, and is associated with incontinence.

Urinary Tract Obstruction

Any type of obstruction in the urinary tract can contribute to urine leakage. Obstructions include bladder stones, tumors, polyps, and other lesions. When the urinary tract is obstructed, it may lead to overflow incontinence. Urinary obstruction can

Rectocele

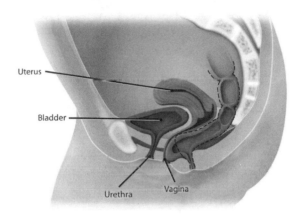

Uterus

Bladder

Urethra

Vagina

Another example of a prolapsed pelvic organ, a rectocele is a prolapse of the rectum. It occurs when the end of the large intestine (rectum) pushes against the back wall of the vagina.

occur in women but it is more commonly seen in men and is typically due to an enlarged prostate.

Genetic Factors

There appears to be a genetic component to incontinence. Studies show that if your mother or sister is incontinent, you have an increased risk of developing the condition as well. One study reported that in patients with incontinence, 23 percent of their mothers and 29 percent of their sisters also had symptoms of the condition. Genetics may also play a role in whether or not you'll experience weakened pelvic muscles due to aging, pregnancy, or childbirth, or thinning pelvic tissues following menopause. Weakened pelvic muscles and thinning pelvic tissues both contribute to incontinence.

Nerve Damage, Neurological Conditions, and Spinal Injuries

Pregnancy, vaginal childbirth, neurological disorders, spinal cord injuries, and pelvic radiation therapy can damage the nerves and muscles that control the bladder and the urethra. Pregnancy and vaginal childbirth are the most common causes of nerve damage. Neurological conditions that may injure pelvic nerves and muscles include multiple sclerosis, Parkinson's disease, stroke, and brain tumors. When the sacral nerves of the bladder are damaged, they may no longer signal the urge to urinate when the bladder is full. In this instance, urine loss may be experienced without any warning or sensation.

Urinary Tract Abnormalities

Urinary tract abnormalities can prevent normal bladder function. For instance, a urogenital fistula is an abnormal opening between the urinary tract and the vagina. This opening allows urine to leak continuously from the vagina. A urogenital fistula is commonly the result of a postoperative healing complication or an erosion of the tissues following radiation therapy for cancer in the pelvic area.

Uncommon Causes of Persistent Incontinence

Interstitial Cystitis

Interstitial cystitis (IC) is a chronic inflammation of the bladder wall that causes painful urination as well as symptoms of urgency and frequency. In severe cases, you may feel the urge to urinate as many as sixty times per day. This condition may also markedly reduce the amount of urine your bladder can hold, contributing to the symptoms of frequency.

More than six hundred thousand women are estimated to have IC, which is far more common in women than in men. Women of all ages can develop IC, but the average age of onset is forty. Although IC can cause symptoms of urgency and frequency, it does not usually lead to the involuntary loss of urine. If you have IC and are incontinent, your incontinence may be due to something other than IC.

Bladder Cancer

In extremely rare cases, incontinence may be a symptom of bladder cancer. Urinary urgency, burning during urination, and blood in the urine may also be signs of bladder cancer. Of course, this condition calls for immediate treatment.

Causes of Temporary Incontinence

There are many causes of temporary incontinence; they are described in the pages that follow. Temporary incontinence is reversible and treatable. In many cases, causes of temporary incontinence are related to your health or to your lifestyle habits.

Pregnancy and Childbirth

Many women experience episodes of incontinence during pregnancy or after childbirth. During pregnancy, the weight of the growing fetus places additional pressure on the bladder, often causing episodes of stress incontinence and symptoms of urgency. With each subsequent pregnancy, you are more likely to develop these temporary symptoms. In many cases, however, your bladder control will be restored some time after childbirth.

Vaginal childbirth increases your risk of developing postpartum stress incontinence. That's because vaginal childbirth causes dramatic stretching and displacement of the pelvic floor structures. In some cases, these damaged muscles, tissues, and nerves don't heal completely and remain weakened. When this is the case, stress incontinence is a common result. Caesarean section procedures are less likely to result in stress incontinence than vaginal births.

Difficult deliveries, such as those involving a large baby, a baby who "gets stuck," or the use of forceps for extraction a baby, may cause increased stress on the support of the bladder. Most urologists agree that these factors may increase a woman's chance of incontinence that persists beyond the healing phase.

In most cases, the damages that occur due to childbirth will eventually heal, and any incontinence you experience following childbirth will only be temporary. However, if your symptoms persist for more than six weeks after delivery, there is a risk that the problem has become one of persistent incontinence.

Infection

Infections that can cause temporary incontinence include urinary tract infections and vaginal infections. A urinary tract infection (UTI) is an infection that occurs anywhere in the urinary tract—the bladder, the urethra, the kidneys, or the ureters. Each year, about 20 percent of women develop a UTI. These infections are commonly caused by bacteria from the anus entering the urethra and then the bladder. You may be at higher risk for developing a UTI if you are pregnant or postmenopausal or if you use a diaphragm for birth control.

When you have a UTI, the infection acts as an irritant, causing inflammation of the bladder and urethral lining. UTIs are characterized by painful urination, frequent urination during the day and night, and sudden urges to urinate. These sudden urges may not give you enough time to get to a bathroom before your bladder empties involuntarily. The urgency symptoms often persist even after you've emptied your bladder, making you feel like you need to go but aren't able to. In some cases, the inflammation of the lining may be so severe that you'll notice blood in your urine. Antibiotics are usually prescribed to treat a UTI and, once you've taken the full course, symptoms typically start to improve within a few days.

Atrophic Urethritis/Vaginitis

These conditions, *atrophic urethritis* and *atrophic vaginitis*, occur as the result of a decrease in estrogen production, typically following menopause. If you have this condition, you may develop symptoms of urgency, frequency, or stress incontinence. In many cases, these hormonal deficits are treatable with estrogen pills or topical estrogen applications. When treated, your symptoms of incontinence may improve considerably.

Pharmaceuticals

Several medications and vitamins can interfere with your ability to control your bladder. For instance, sedatives can slow your ability to react to the urge to urinate. Antidepressants, antianxiety pills, and muscle relaxants cause a relaxation of the bladder muscle. This may contribute to overflow incontinence. Decongestants for the common cold have the opposite effect on the urethra, causing it to constrict. This may bring on a sense of urgency and may lead to overflow incontinence.

Diuretics, also called water pills, tend to increase frequency and urgency, sometimes resulting in accidents. Some medications for heart conditions, irritable bowel syndrome, and Parkinson's disease decrease the bladder's ability to signal when it is full. Asthma medications and high doses of vitamin C, vitamin B, or calcium can act as bladder irritants. The good news is that your symptoms of frequency, urgency, or involuntary loss of urine should disappear when you stop taking these medications or vitamins. Be sure to consult with your doctor before stopping any prescribed medications.

Excess Output

An increase in urine output, also known as *polyuria*, is commonly associated with symptoms of urgency, frequency, and involuntary loss of urine. Several medical conditions and medications can induce excess urine production. Conditions include hyperglycemia (increased blood sugar), increased blood calcium, congestive heart failure, chronic leg edema, lower extremity venous insufficiency, and diabetes. Medications that increase urine production are called diuretics or water pills and are often used to treat heart failure, high blood pressure, kidney diseases, and liver disease. Seeking treatment for these medical conditions or eliminating these medications from your daily regimen may put a halt to incontinence. Of course, you should always check with your physician before stopping any medication.

Medications that May Affect Bladder Control

Type of Medication	Effect	Symptoms
Antianxiety/muscle relaxants Antiseizure medications	Relaxation of the bladder muscle	Overflow
Decongestants	Constriction of the urethra	Urgency Overflow
Anticholinergics Calcium blockers	Decreased bladder sensation and Decreased muscle tone	Overflow
Vitamin C (high doses) Vitamin B (high doses) Calcium (high doses) Asthma medications	Irritates and stimulates the bladder	Frequency Urgency
Constipation medications Cough medicines	Increases pressure on the bladder	Frequency Urgency
Diuretics	Increases urine production	Frequency Urgency Overflow

Restricted Mobility

When you aren't able to get to the bathroom or get your clothes off quickly when you have an urge to urinate, it can lead to situational incontinence. Restricted mobility is most commonly seen in senior adults who have arthritis or who are otherwise impaired, but it can also affect younger women. For instance, if you've suffered an injury or you've undergone surgery, you may not be able to move around as swiftly as usual. Once you recover, your bladder control should return to normal.

Stool Impaction

Constipation that results in impacted stool—a large mass of dry, hard stool in the rectum—can cause bladder control problems. The pressure from the stool can obstruct the flow of urine and may prevent the bladder from emptying completely. This can result in episodes of overflow incontinence or urge incontinence. Stool impaction may also lead to urinary frequency and urgency and is considered to be a fairly common cause of temporary incontinence.

Dehydration

Dehydration can bring on bladder problems. When you don't take in adequate amounts of fluid, your urine becomes very concentrated. The concentrated urine may act as a bladder irritant, creating a constant urge to urinate. Once your fluid levels are returned to normal, your urination patterns should also return to normal. Try to drink four to eight eight-ounce glasses of fluid per day to stay hydrated.

Retention

Increased urinary retention can produce difficulty urinating, the inability to completely empty the bladder, and episodes of stress or urge incontinence. Urinary retention may be the result of depression, pelvic surgery, or even surgery performed to correct incontinence.

Psychiatric disorders

Psychological problems don't directly cause incontinence. However, they may indirectly have an effect on bladder control. For instance, if you suffer from depression, you may not feel like participating in your normal physical activities. Decreased activity levels may increase fluid retention, which can create unpredictable needs to urinate, stress incontinence, and urge incontinence. Depression can also lead to abnormal eating behavior, increasing your chances of becoming obese, which places additional pressure on the bladder. Anxiety and emotional stress are known to increase bladder activity, contributing to urge sensations and sometimes incontinence.

If you seek help for psychological problems, you may notice that your symptoms of incontinence improve as your mental health improves. However, some medicines can also contribute to incontinence. Lithium, a drug prescribed to control bipolar disorder, acts as a diuretic, causing urgency and frequency.

Other diseases that affect mental acuity, such as Alzheimer's, can lead to accidents. For instance, Alzheimer's patients may not be able to react to the need to urinate quickly enough, or may not remember how to get to the bathroom.

Delirium

Delirium refers to a strong sense of disorientation or mental confusion. This may develop as the result of a serious illness or from a severe lack of sleep. Certain medications and anesthesia can also produce delirium in some people. When you're in a state of delirium, you may not be aware of the need to urinate, or you may not be able to react in time to avoid an accident. Your bladder control should return to normal once the cause of your delirium has passed.

Fluid Intake

Normal urine production depends on normal fluid intake. Drinking more fluids than your body needs can have a negative affect on bladder function. For instance, drinking large amounts of water or any other fluid—especially in a short amount of time—increases urine production. When this occurs, the bladder must deal with the increase in urine, which can cause symptoms of urgency, frequency, and even incontinence. In addition, a rapid intake of fluids can overload your bladder, causing it to fill beyond its capacity. In this case, you may even experience backflow or reflux, in which the urine flows back from the bladder toward the kidneys. Symptoms of this would be continuous overflow incontinence, leading to kidney filtering problems and infections. Your doctor will want to identify the cause of the reflux in order to determine the best treatment.

Foods and Beverages that May Act as Irritants or Diuretics

Alcohol	Apple Juice	Apples
Apricots	Artificial sweeteners	Asparagus
Avocados	BBQ sauce	Bananas
Beets	Cabbage	Caffeinated beverages
Cantaloupe	Carbonated sodas	Cheese (except American, cottage, ricotta, & cream)
Chicken liver	Chilies	Chocolate
Citrus fruits	Citrus juices	Cocktail sauce
Corned beef	Corn syrup	Cranberries
Cucumbers	Grapefruit	Guava
Honey	Ketchup	Lemons
Lentils	Lima beans	Mayonnaise
Milk and milk products	Mustard	Onions
Peaches	Pickled herring	Pickles
Plums	Prunes	Raisins
Relish	Rhubarb	Rye bread
Sauerkraut	Sour cream	Soy sauce
Spicy foods	Strawberries	Sugar
Tomato-based products	Vinegar	Watermelon
Yogurt		

Foods and Beverages

A number of foods and beverages can cause temporary cases of urgency, frequency, or the involuntary loss of urine. For instance, some foods and beverages act as a *diuretic*. A diuretic is something that increases urine production and causes your bladder to fill more quickly than usual. In some cases, this may trigger a sudden urge to urinate, sometimes so sudden that you don't have time to get to the bathroom. Fluids that fall into this category include alcohol, caffeinated beverages, such as coffee, tea, and caffeinated sodas.

Other foods and beverages can irritate the bladder. Spicy foods, carbonated sodas, citrus juices, and artificial sweeteners are considered common irritants. For most women, these foods and beverages cause no problem. However, in a few people, they create what's often described as a "prickly sensation" in the bladder that leads to an urge to urinate. Alcoholic beverages pose other problems. First, as a diuretic, alcohol causes increased urine production; excessive use of alcohol causes sedation, altered sensory awareness, and impaired mobility, it can reduce your ability to recognize and act on the need to urinate in a timely fashion.

Smoking

Smoking affects your ability to control your bladder in a number of ways. For example, many smokers experience a chronic cough, which places extra pressure on the bladder, the pelvic floor, and the urethra. These external pressures contribute to pelvic organ prolapse and stress incontinence. In addition, nicotine acts as a bladder irritant, which can cause urge incontinence. In fact, smokers are twice as likely to develop symptoms of urge incontinence than nonsmokers.

Smoking also raises your risk of developing bladder cancer and cancer of the lining of the urethra. Both of these conditions can lead to incontinence. If you smoke twenty or more cigarettes per day, all of these risks are more pronounced. Quitting smoking may reverse these effects and restore your ability to control your bladder.

Going to the Bathroom "Just in Case..."

If you regularly use the bathroom "just in case you need to go later," even though you don't really have to urinate, you could be headed for bladder trouble. Millions of women fall into this category. If you're one of them, you may find that you always use the bathroom before leaving the house, or that you stop in every public restroom you come across because you aren't sure when you'll find another one. Basically, what you're doing is training your bladder to empty when it isn't full. Ultimately, your bladder learns to signal the urge to urinate even when it hasn't reached its capacity. This may increase your chance of developing symptoms of frequency, urgency, and even incontinence.

Bathroom habits such as these are often an occupational hazard. Teachers, nurses, factory workers, truck drivers, and pilots often work without easy access to a bathroom. When a bathroom is available, they tend to use it even if they don't really need to. Urinating more frequently than you need to can result in a gradual decrease in the amount of urine the bladder can comfortably hold.

The opposite extreme of this habit is holding your urine for many hours at a time, and this can also cause problems. It can gradually stretch the bladder until it's injured from overstretching. If this occurs, your bladder may become desensitized, meaning it won't signal you with the urge to urinate when it is full.

Leaking during Exercise

Engaging in high-impact sports and activities may bring on temporary episodes of stress incontinence. These activities place extra pressure on your bladder, which causes leakage in some women. However, this type of incontinence is considered situational and typically disappears once you stop the activity. Sports and activities that may lead to leakage include:

- High-impact aerobics
- Racket sports
- Jogging
- Marathon running
- Hiking
- Distance walking

Lack of Physical Activity

A general lack of physical activity may contribute to the weakening of the muscles of the pelvic floor and subsequently may cause stress incontinence. Studies show that exercising—even at a low level of intensity—for as little as an hour each week can lower your risk of developing incontinence. Starting an exercise routine may help eliminate any symptoms you have. Always consult your family doctor or primary care physician prior to starting an exercise program.

Being Overweight

If you're overweight or obese, you may be at greater risk for incontinence. Some reports estimate that 63 percent of obese patients experience stress incontinence and an additional 27 percent suffer from symptoms of urge incontinence. Why is incontinence so prevalent in the obese? The extra weight of the abdomen places additional pressure on the bladder and weakens the muscles of the pelvic floor. When the bladder and surrounding muscles are weakened, there's a higher chance of experiencing leakage.

If you're obese, you may also suffer from sleep apnea, a condition in which your breathing stops while you are sleeping. Typically, the pauses in breathing range from about twenty to thirty seconds each and may occur as many as twenty to thirty times per night. Approximately 60 to 70 percent of obese people are estimated to have sleep apnea. This condition has been associated with an increased need to get up several times a night to urinate. This is called nocturia. Sleep apnea can also contribute to an increased risk of bed-wetting and daytime symptoms of urgency and frequency. Losing weight can alleviate your symptoms.

Cold Temperatures

Cold winter temperatures may play a role in occasional episodes of incontinence. For instance, if you go from inside a warm house into the cold outdoors, you may experience a sense of urgency. This can also occur if you sit on an icy cold bench. This type of situational incontinence usually does not develop into a chronic problem.

Chapter 3

Getting a Diagnosis

I f your incontinence has persisted, you should be checked out by a physician. You're probably wondering how your doctor will arrive at a diagnosis. Actually, there are several tests he or she may perform to determine which type of incontinence you have and what may be causing it. In many cases, a simple physical exam and a few basic tests are all that is needed to make a diagnosis. In other instances, more-advanced testing may be necessary to discover what is causing your incontinence. No matter what type of incontinence you have, you can help ensure a proper diagnosis by providing your physician with as much information as possible about your symptoms.

■ Which kind of doctor should I see for help with incontinence?

For an initial evaluation, consider making an appointment with your primary care physician or gynecologist. Because you probably already have a rapport with this person, you'll likely feel more comfortable discussing your symptoms. In many cases, a family doctor, primary care physician, or gynecologist will be able to diagnose and treat your incontinence.

In some cases, however, you may prefer to go directly to an incontinence specialist, or your doctor may recommend that you see a specialist, such as a *urologist* or a *urogynecologist*. A urologist is a doctor who specializes in urinary disorders in both women and men as well as in the male reproductive system. A urogynecologist is an obstetrician/gynecologist who specializes in the care of women with pelvic floor dysfunction, including urinary incontinence.

If you need help finding a specialist, you may want to ask your primary care physician or a trusted friend or family member. You can also find incontinence specialists on a number of reputable Web sites, such as the American Urological Association Foundation (www.urologyhealth.com), the National Institute of Diabetes and Digestive and Kidney Diseases (kidney.niddk.nih.gov), and the American Urogynecologic Society Foundation (www.augs.org). Whether you choose to see a primary care physician or a specialist, your doctor should take the time to answer all of your questions about incontinence.

■ **Do most women with incontinence seek help?**

The vast majority of women with incontinence do not seek help for the problem. In fact, studies estimate that only one in twelve women with incontinence go to a medical professional for help. In many cases, they may be too ashamed to seek help, or they may not realize that incontinence can be treated. But there are treatments available, and consulting a doctor about the problem is an important first step in improving the situation.

Most of the women who seek help only do so after they've been experiencing symptoms of incontinence for several years. Often, there's a specific event that spurs a visit to a physician—usually leaking urine in a social setting or avoiding an important social occasion due to fear of an accident. In most cases, the sooner you seek help, the sooner you'll be able to take control of your bladder and your life.

■ **What if I'm too embarrassed to talk about this problem with a doctor?**

If you feel too embarrassed to discuss your symptoms with your doctor, remember that incontinence is a medical problem—the same way heart disease is a medical problem or breaking your arm is a medical problem. In some instances, incontinence may be a symptom of a more serious underlying condition. This makes it even more important for you to discuss the problem with your doctor.

Remember that incontinence isn't your fault, and your doctor isn't going to judge you or think less of you because this is happening to you. In addition, keep in mind that incontinence is a very common problem affecting millions of women. It's very likely your physician has already evaluated and treated many other women who experience urinary leakage.

■ How should I prepare for a visit with the doctor?

In most cases, you don't need to do anything special to prepare for an evaluation. However, it is a good idea to jot down some notes about your medical history. Things you may want to include are:

- Pregnancies
- Vaginal deliveries
- Date you entered menopause, if applicable
- Pelvic operations
- Injuries to the pelvic area
- Health conditions
- Mental health disorders

In addition, make a list of all the medications you're currently taking, including prescription drugs, over-the-counter medications, vitamins, and supplements. Write down the dosage of each medication and the frequency with which you take it. Some doctors will ask you to bring your medications with you to your first appointment. By taking a look at your medications, your physician can determine if any of them may be a possible cause for your incontinence.

For a few days prior to your visit, you may also be asked to keep a record of the number of times you leak and the volume of leakage—for example, a few drops or completely soaking through a pad. This record is referred to as a voiding diary.

In addition to recording information about leakage, a voiding diary may also include a record of your activities, fluid intake, the number of times you urinate, and the amount of urgency you experience.

■ What should I expect during an evaluation?

During an initial evaluation, your doctor will ask about your urinary complaints and your lifestyle habits, will take down a thorough medical history, and will perform a physical exam. He or she will also perform a few routine tests. If you have prepared a voiding diary, your physician will review it with you to get a better understanding of your problem.

When discussing your incontinence and your medical history, try to be as thorough as possible. Don't leave anything out because you aren't sure whether or not it is significant. Something you think is unimportant may actually be the cause of your urinary troubles. By giving your doctor all the information you can, you will help him or her reach a proper diagnosis.

■ What are some questions commonly asked by urologists?

Your doctor will ask you a variety of questions to zero in on a diagnosis. You can expect to answer questions about your urologic history and complaints, about your lifestyle habits, and about your quality of life. In some cases, he or she may also ask you "environmental" questions, which focus on the layout of your home and your furnishings. Many specialists will have you fill out a questionnaire that is designed specifically to help determine which type of incontinence you have and how much it is affecting your life. Specialists may send you a questionnaire and ask you to fill it out before coming to your appointment, or you may be asked to fill out a questionnaire when you arrive at the office for your appointment.

Urological Questions

You can expect to be asked numerous questions about your urinary habits and complaints. Here is a list of questions you may be asked regarding your urologic health.

- What is your most troubling urinary problem?
- How long has this been taking place?
- Are your symptoms getting worse, improving, or staying the same?
- After urinating, does your bladder feel empty, or do you feel like you still have urine in your bladder?
- Do you continue to drip a few drops of urine after you've finished urinating?
- How many times do you urinate during the day?
- How many times do you urinate during the night?
- Do you urinate more often than you need to in order to prevent an accident?
- Do you have difficulty starting the urine stream?
- While urinating, is the flow continuous, or does it start and stop?
- Is the force of the stream strong, weak, or fair?
- When there is a strong desire to urinate, can it be postponed?
- What is the longest amount of time you can hold your bladder?
- When there is a strong urge, is there leakage before you reach the toilet?
- Do you leak without realizing it?
- Which activities cause you to leak urine? (For instance, sneezing, coughing, laughing, lifting, running, standing up from a sitting position, bending down, reaching up, washing hands,

seeing or hearing running water, unlocking the front door, walking to the bathroom, sexual activity, being out in cold weather.)

- If there is leakage, what do you use to protect your clothing?
- Do you use this protection during the day and/or at night?
- How many times do you change your pads each day?
- When you change them, are the pads dry, soaked, or moist?
- Do you wet the bed while you sleep?
- Do you get repeated urinary infections?
- Do you experience pain when you urinate?
- Have you ever noticed blood in your urine?
- Do you feel bulging or a protrusion in the vaginal area?
- Do you have constipation?

These questions can assist your doctor in determining which type of incontinence you have as well as the severity of your problem.

Lifestyle Questions

Your doctor may also ask you several questions about your lifestyle and dietary habits. For instance, you may be asked the following questions:

- Do you smoke?
- Have you ever smoked?
- If so, when did you begin smoking?
- If you currently smoke, how many cigarettes do you smoke each day?
- If you've stopped smoking, when did you stop?

■ Do you drink alcoholic beverages, and if so, how many ounces per day?

■ Do you drink caffeinated beverages, and if so, how many ounces per day?

■ Do you drink carbonated sodas, and if so, how many ounces per day?

■ Do you drink beverages with artificial sweeteners, and if so, how many ounces per day?

■ What is your level of physical activity?

These lifestyle and dietary questions can help your physician determine whether the foods and beverages you consume or your activity level are playing a role in your incontinence.

Quality-of-Life Questions

To understand how much of an effect urinary incontinence is having on your quality of life, you may be asked to fill out a questionnaire called the Incontinence Impact Questionnaire. This questionnaire includes questions about your physical activities, your social activities and relationships, your ability to travel, and your emotional health. Questions included on the Incontinence Impact Questionnaire include:

■ Has urine leakage affected your ability to do household chores, such as cooking, laundry, or housecleaning?

■ Has urine leakage affected your physical recreation, such as walking, swimming, or other exercise?

■ Has urine leakage affected your entertainment activities, such as going to the movies or concerts?

■ Has urine leakage affected your ability to travel by car or bus more than thirty minutes from home?

■ Has urine leakage affected your participation in social activities outside your home?

- Has urine leakage affected your emotional health, causing nervousness, depression, etc.?
- Has urine leakage left you feeling frustrated?

The Incontinence Impact Questionnaire asks you to rate to what degree urinary leakage has affected your life in each of these areas: not at all, slightly, moderately, or greatly. With your responses to these questions, your doctor will have a much clearer picture of your individual experience with incontinence.

Environmental Questions

In some cases, the design of your home, your furnishings, or your clothing may be to blame for some of your accidents. To determine if your home or clothing creates obstacles for you, your physician may ask some of the following questions.

- Is your bathroom easily accessible from your bedroom?
- Do you need to climb any steps to get to your bathroom?
- Do you have difficulty rising out of the chairs in your home?
- Do you have grab bars in your bathroom to assist you with sitting and standing?
- Do you have difficulty undoing buttons or zippers in a timely fashion?

Based on your answers to these questions, your doctor may determine that you have functional incontinence. Many times, simple changes to your home or in the type of clothing you wear can reduce or even eliminate urinary accidents.

- **What is involved in the physical exam?**

A physical exam for an initial evaluation is typically painless. An exam usually involves a limited pelvic exam, a brief rectal exam, and an abdominal exam. In some cases, your physician may also perform an assessment of your mobility, a neurologic exam, and a check for any signs of swelling in your legs.

The Physical Exam

Pelvic Exam

A pelvic exam can alert your physician to several potential causes of incontinence, including thinning genital tissues, abnormal nerve responses, pelvic organ prolapse, pelvic floor muscle weakness, and infection. When your physician is ready to begin the exam, he or she will ask you to lie down on an exam table and to put your feet up in stirrups. Your doctor may begin with an external evaluation of your genitals, looking for signs of dryness, redness, or thinning tissues.

A quick test may be performed to assess whether the sacral nerves in your genital area are functioning properly. These nerves play an important role in normal urination by telling you when it is time to urinate. If the nerves are damaged, you may not be receiving the proper signals to alert you when your bladder is full. This nerve test may involve using a cotton swab to touch the areas around your vagina and anus. Your ability to feel each touch will be noted. Other methods may be used to test these nerves. If your nerves don't respond to these tests in a normal way, it could indicate that nerve damage is contributing to your incontinence.

To begin your internal pelvic exam, your physician may simply insert one or two gloved fingers into your vagina. This allows the doctor to feel your bladder and to determine if your pelvic organs are positioned correctly or if they may be bulging into the vaginal wall. This would be a sign of pelvic organ prolapse, which occurs when pelvic structures, such as the bladder or rectum, drop from their normal position and protrude into the vaginal wall. Pelvic organ prolapse is often associated with incontinence.

While your doctor's fingers are inside your vagina, you may be asked to cough or strain so that he or she can evaluate the strength or weakness of your pelvic floor muscles. Your physician can also feel for any masses within the pelvic area. In some instances, a medical instrument called a speculum may be inserted into your vagina to allow the physician to get a better view of your pelvic tissues. He or she can check if these tissues appear to be thinning or if you have any signs of a vaginal infection, such as discharge or inflammation.

Rectal Exam

A brief rectal exam, in which the doctor inserts a gloved finger into the rectum, may be part of your evaluation. Although a bit uncomfortable, a rectal exam should be painless. It can reveal the presence of any masses or an impacted stool, which is commonly linked to incontinence. As mentioned earlier, an impacted stool is a dry, hard mass that develops in the rectum due to chronic constipation. By asking you to squeeze your anal muscles during this portion of the exam, your doctor can test the strength of your pelvic floor muscles.

Abdominal Exam

An abdominal exam can help your physician estimate the size of your bladder, identify any abnormal growths, and look for signs of constipation. To perform an abdominal exam, your doctor will simply press on your abdomen with his or her hands. While pushing on the bladder area, your doctor will be checking to see if your bladder feels larger than usual or if you feel any pain or discomfort. An enlarged bladder and soreness are sometimes associated with overflow incontinence.

By feeling your abdomen, your physician can also detect tumors, hernias, and other growths that may play a part in your incontinence. While pressing on your abdomen, your doctor may also be listening for normal bowel sounds. If there are no bowel sounds, it could be an indication of constipation. Chronic constipation can lead to impacted stool, which is a common cause of incontinence.

Mobility Exam

The purpose of a mobility exam is to assess your ability to walk, sit, and stand up, and to evaluate your manual dexterity. To assess your mobility, your doctor may simply observe your movement during the appointment. If you demonstrate signs of limited mobility, such as having trouble maneuvering yourself onto the exam table or having trouble rising from a seated position, this could indicate that you have functional incontinence.

Neurologic Exam

If your physician suspects that you may have a neurologic problem, a neurologic exam may be performed. This can help determine if your nerves are functioning normally, or if you may have nerve damage. The neurologic exam is performed using a reflex hammer and, in some cases, a sharp pin. Typically, your doctor will tap your legs in various spots to test your reflexes. He or she may then touch your legs with the reflex hammer and a sharp pin and ask you if you can differentiate between the two. If you aren't able to tell the difference or if your reflexes don't respond normally, it could indicate that a neurologic problem is contributing to your incontinence.

Lower Extremity Exam

A lower extremity exam is performed to determine if an underlying disease may be to blame for your incontinence. Your doctor may check your legs, ankles, and feet for any signs of swelling. If you have swelling in your lower extremities, it could be a sign of an underlying condition, such as diabetes, congestive heart failure, or kidney disease. When swelling is present, it can lead to urinary incontinence—especially at night. That's because when you lie down in bed, the excess fluids in your lower extremities are absorbed by the body and processed through the bladder. This typically results in increased urine production, which may lead to accidents.

Diagnostic Tests

An initial evaluation usually includes only a few simple, painless tests—there are no biopsies and no catheters required. These tests may include a stress test, a routine urinalysis, and a blood test. To perform a stress test, your doctor may ask you to cough, walk around, jump up and down, or bend over. If you leak during this test, you may have stress incontinence.

For a urinalysis, you'll be asked to urinate in a small cup provided by your doctor. The urine is then tested for bacteria, which could indicate a urinary tract infection, which is a common cause of temporary incontinence. Your doctor may draw your blood to test it for a variety of chemicals and other substances that may contribute to incontinence.

In many cases, your doctor will be able to make a diagnosis based on these tests, on your physical exam, and on the information you've provided. If the tests are inconclusive, additional testing may be required.

■ Is ultrasound used to diagnose incontinence?

Ultrasound may be used as part of routine testing to diagnose incontinence. Your doctor will usually perform an ultrasound after you've urinated, to assess the amount of residual urine in the bladder. Many healthy women will have some urine remaining in the bladder after urinating. However, if you have a large amount of urine left over in the bladder, it could be a sign of overflow incontinence. Excessive urine remaining in the bladder could also indicate a blockage in your urinary tract, a nerve problem, or a dysfunctional bladder muscle.

An ultrasound to diagnose incontinence is performed by applying a gel on the lower abdomen and passing a wand back and forth over the abdomen. It is not a vaginal ultrasound in which a wand is inserted into the vagina. The device sends sound waves through the abdominal area, and a computer transforms these sound waves into images that can be viewed on a monitor. On the monitor, your doctor will be able to see the amount of urine remaining in your bladder. The procedure is noninvasive, and you can return to your normal activities or go back to work when it has been completed.

■ How do doctors determine how much leakage is being experienced?

Doctors often use a *pad test* to help determine how much urinary leakage you're experiencing. This test involves wearing protective pads designed for urinary incontinence. If you normally wear protective pads, your doctor may ask you to keep a record of how many times a day you need to change your pads and how wet the pads are when you change them.

In some cases, your doctor may have you wear a pad while you're in the doctor's office and then he or she will examine it to see how much moisture has been soaked up. In other cases, your doctor may send you home with some pads. You'll wear the pads for a prescribed amount of time and then seal them in plastic bags that you take back to the doctor's office where they are weighed. This last method provides the most accurate measure of the amount of urine that's leaking.

■ What is cystoscopy and is it part of an initial evaluation?

Cystoscopy is a procedure that allows a doctor to see inside your bladder and urethra using a *cystoscope*—a long, thin instrument with a tiny camera on the tip. This test is not included in a routine evaluation. Instead, it may be recommended if you don't respond to initial treatments, if you have had recurring urinary tract infections, if you have blood in the urine, if you have a neurological disease, or if surgery to correct incontinence has failed. Cystoscopy is also routinely performed prior to having surgery to treat incontinence. If you require a cystoscopy, you will likely be referred to a specialist, such as a urologist or urogynecologist.

The procedure involves the insertion of a small telescope into the urethra and up into the bladder. With this device, your doctor can see the bladder and check for infection, inflammation, tumors, bladder stones, or abnormal variations in anatomy. With the scope in place, your doctor can also biopsy any polyps or growths.

Cystoscopy is an office-based procedure that takes only about five minutes. An antibiotic may be given to reduce the risk of infection. If you are feeling anxious about the procedure, your doctor may give you a sedative to help you relax. The procedure is performed while you are lying on your back, often with your feet in stirrups. Your urethra is cleaned with an antiseptic, and a numbing gel may be used to minimize discomfort. Next, the thin tubelike telescope is gently guided into the urethra and then into the bladder. Your doctor may look directly into the end of the scope, or the image may be projected onto a small television screen. Once your doctor has evaluated your bladder and urethra, the scope is removed.

After your procedure, you may experience a minor stinging or burning sensation in the urethra. This usually lasts until the next time you urinate, but in some cases, it may last a bit longer. Typically, there are no restrictions on your activities following cystoscopy; however, your doctor may recommend that you go home and rest for the remainder of the day. If sedation was used, you won't be allowed to drive following the procedure, so you'll need to arrange for someone to take you home.

■ What is urodynamic testing and when is it recommended?

Urodynamic testing (UDT) is a sophisticated series of tests that lets your doctor evaluate your bladder in action. This test is routinely performed preoperatively if you are going to have surgery to treat incontinence. It may also be recommended if you don't respond to first-line therapy, if you have a neurological disease, or if surgery to correct incontinence has failed. Urodynamic testing is usually performed by specialists in urinary dysfunction, including urologists and urogynecologists.

The series of tests takes less than an hour and may be performed either in your doctor's office or in an outpatient facility. In general, you don't need to do anything in particular to prepare for the procedure, although you may be asked to arrive with a full bladder. Tests that may be included in your UDT include uroflowmetry and cystometry.

Uroflowmetry: This test measures how fast or how slowly your urine comes out. In this test, you simply urinate into a special receptacle that calculates the pattern and force of your stream.

Cystometry: This test measures the pressure in your bladder when it's empty, as it fills, and while you are urinating. With your bladder empty, you'll be asked to lie down on an examination table. Your genital area will be cleansed with antiseptic to prevent infection, and a numbing gel is commonly applied to reduce any painful sensations. A very thin catheter will be gently inserted into your urethra and up into your bladder. You may feel a slight pinch or sting as the catheter is inserted. When the catheter is in place, a separate catheter may be placed in your vagina. The catheters, which are connected to computers, are taped in place.

You may be asked to stand or sit to begin the test. The catheter is used to slowly fill your bladder with sterile water. As your bladder is filled, the computers record the pressure within your bladder. Your doctor may ask you about the sensations you are feeling, and may ask you to cough at various times during the test to see if you leak. The pressure at which you leak urine is called the *leak point pressure.*

Your doctor will stop filling your bladder when you feel that it is full and that you need to urinate. With the catheters still in place, you'll be asked to urinate into a special container. As you urinate, pressure changes in the bladder and urethra will be recorded. This is called a *voiding study.* After you've urinated, the catheter will be slowly removed from your urethra in order to test the urethra's ability to close. This is called a *urethral pressure profile.*

At some point during UDT, your doctor may also perform a *postvoid residual test.* This test measures how much urine is left in the bladder after you've urinated. After you've urinated, the doctor will drain the remaining urine from your bladder using the catheter. After this portion of the test is completed, the catheters are typically removed and the test is over.

In some instances, your doctor may also take X-rays of your bladder during the filling and voiding portions of the test. In this procedure, rather than using sterile water to fill your bladder, your doctor will use a clear fluid that appears white on X-ray. This fluid is harmless because it only comes in contact with your bladder and doesn't enter your bloodstream. This procedure is called a *video urodynamics study* or a *cystogram*. The video can pinpoint blockages in the urinary tract and can reveal whether the bladder and urethra are working properly or if they are opening or contracting at inappropriate times.

Following urodynamic testing, you may experience a stinging sensation in the urethra. The burning usually only lasts until the next time you urinate, but in some cases, the unpleasant sensation may last a bit longer. You may also feel the need to urinate more frequently and may experience an increased sense of urgency. In some cases, you may notice a small amount of blood discoloration in your urine. This generally occurs if there was some resistance while inserting the catheter in the urethra and isn't a cause for concern. After your UDT, there are no restrictions on your activities. You can return to work, or you can go home if you prefer to rest for the remainder of the day.

■ **Is it ever necessary to perform tests that help the doctor see the kidneys as well as the bladder?**

In cases of overflow incontinence, it may be beneficial for your doctor to be able to view your kidneys in addition to your bladder. As explained previously, severe cases of overflow incontinence may result in urine flowing from the bladder back to the kidneys. If this occurs, it may lead to problems with the kidneys.

Patient name:

Intake & Voiding Diary

✍✍ *This chart is a record of your fluid intake, voiding, and urine leakage.*

✍✍ *Choose 4 days (entire 24 hours) to complete this record— they DO NOT have to be in a row.*

✍✍ *Pick days in which will be convenient for you to measure EVERY void.*

✍✍ *Please take this diary to your next visit.*

INSTRUCTIONS:

1. Begin recording upon rising in the morning—continue for a full 24 hours.
2. Record separate times for voids, leaks, and fluid intake.
3. Measure voids in "ccs" using the hat.
4. Measure fluid intake in ounces.
5. When recording a leak—please indicate the volume ("1,2, or 3"), your activity during the leak, and if you had an urge ("yes" or "no").

Examples of entries

TIME	Amount voided (in ccs)	LEAK Volume 1 = drops/damp 2 = wet-soaked 3 = bladder emptied	Activity during leak	Was there an urge?	Fluid intake (Amount in ounces/type)
7:00a	250 cc	2	Running	Yes	
7:30a					8 oz./Herbal tea

TIME	Amount voided (in ccs)	LEAK Volume 1 = drops/damp 2 = wet-soaked 3 = bladder emptied	Activity during leak	Was there an urge?	Fluid intake (Amount in ounces/type)

Source: American Urogynecologic Society Foundation

To get a look at your kidneys, your physician may use ultrasound, as described previously, or a CT scan. A CT scan is a painless, noninvasive test that uses special X-ray equipment to take images of your body. CT scanners are typically large machines with a hole in the center and an examination table that moves through the hole.

For a CT exam, you will be asked to lie down on the table, and the X-rays will rotate around you. In some cases, an iodine dye may be injected into a vein in your arm or taken orally to enhance the visibility of the kidneys. When dye is used, you may be asked to fast for a certain period of time prior to your exam. The CT scan usually takes only a few minutes. When your scan is completed, you can return to your normal activities.

■ What is the Q-Tip test?

A Q-Tip test may be performed to determine if you have stress incontinence. In this test, a common Q-Tip covered with numbing gel is inserted into the urethra while you are lying down with your feet in stirrups. You are asked to cough and strain. While you do so, the doctor measures the angle of the end of the Q-Tip. If the angle of the Q-Tip changes excessively, it may indicate stress incontinence. This test used to be a common part of routine evaluations for incontinence, but it is rarely used today because more-sophisticated testing options are now available.

■ How do I use a voiding diary, and how does it help a doctor make a diagnosis?

Your physician may ask you to keep a voiding diary following your first appointment. A voiding diary is used to keep track of when you urinate, when you feel urgency, when you leak, how much you leak, and what activity—if any—triggered the leakage. You can also use a voiding diary to keep track of your fluid intake, recording what you drink, how much you drink, and when you drink it. In your diary, you can also record how many times a day you need to change your pads, if you use protection.

This written diary is an important tool that may assist your doctor in diagnosing which type of incontinence you have, what's causing it, and how much it is affecting your life. It is typically far more accurate than simply relying on your memory to inform your doctor about your bladder control problems.

A voiding diary doesn't have to be fancy. You can simply keep track in a regular notebook, or your doctor may have a sample voiding diary that you can use. You can also download a voiding diary free of charge at the American Urogynecologic Society Foundation Web site (www.augs.org).

■ How long will it take to get a diagnosis?

In most cases, you will leave your initial evaluation with a diagnosis. If you require additional testing, such as cystoscopy or urodynamic studies, you'll have the results of those tests immediately. There's no waiting for your doctor to send your tests out to a lab. Your results can be viewed and discussed during your appointment. Based on your results, a diagnosis can be established.

■ Do insurance companies cover the costs of these tests?

All of the tests used for diagnosing incontinence are covered by insurance and Medicare. Depending on your insurer and your particular health plan, you may be responsible for paying a deductible or for a portion of the costs.

■ Do most women who seek help overcome incontinence?

The vast majority of women who seek help for incontinence see an improvement in their situation. This is why you should discuss your symptoms with your doctor. The simple act of making an appointment could help you do far more than regain control of your bladder. It may also be the first step in allowing you to participate once again in your favorite activities, in bolstering your self-esteem, and in enjoying your social life.

Part II

Treatments for Incontinence

Chapter 4

Lifestyle Changes and Exercises

You may be pleasantly surprised to discover that there are some very simple things you can do that may treat incontinence. In fact, treating your incontinence may require nothing more than a few changes in your lifestyle or a few easy exercises to strengthen your pelvic floor muscles. These types of treatments are called behavioral therapies, and depending on your diagnosis, many doctors prescribe them as a first line of treatment. Behavioral therapies can be very effective, cause no side effects, and usually don't cost anything. This makes them very popular with both doctors and patients.

Of course, lifestyle changes and exercises don't solve every case of incontinence. In some instances, behavioral therapy may be recommended in tandem with other types of treatment to boost their healing power. At other times, they may be recommended before turning to more-invasive types of treatment.

Fortunately, there is a wide variety of simple things you can do that may improve your situation. Behavioral therapies that may have a beneficial effect on symptoms of incontinence include simple changes in your diet, bladder retraining, and pelvic floor muscle exercises. Depending on the type and severity of your incontinence, your doctor may recommend that you try one type of behavioral therapy or several approaches at the same time.

It is important that you understand that behavioral therapies require a commitment on your part. You must be willing to take the time to perform any recommended exercises, and you must put forth a concerted effort to make changes to your lifestyle. In some cases, changing lifelong habits may prove to be more difficult than you expected. But if you don't do your part, you won't see any improvements in your symptoms. Keep this in mind if your doctor suggests behavioral therapies as a treatment option. On the plus side, behavioral therapy usually doesn't cost a thing and is safe to do.

■ Is it beneficial to change the kinds of beverages I drink?

In most cases, it can be beneficial to change the types of fluids you consume. As mentioned previously, beverages that act as diuretics or that irritate the bladder can cause incontinence. Fluids that act as diuretics include caffeinated and alcoholic beverages. Bladder irritants include coffee, tea, acidic fruit juices, and carbonated sodas. Replacing these types of beverages with water or other nonirritating drinks can be helpful in reducing symptoms of urgency and urinary leakage.

For instance, if you drink several cups of coffee a day, gradually taper your intake and then stop drinking all coffee for a while. Some doctors may recommend cutting it out for a matter of days; others may suggest avoiding it for a few weeks. If your symptoms improve, you may want to cut coffee out of your diet completely. If you don't notice any improvement after avoiding coffee for the prescribed amount of time, your doctor may advise you that you can add it back to your daily routine.

In some cases, eliminating one beverage at a time can help you pinpoint the specific fluids that irritate your bladder and trigger your symptoms. If you drink carbonated sodas, citrus juices, and coffee, try restricting one of them first. For example, eliminate your intake of sodas for the amount of time recommended by your doctor. If there's no change, add it back to your diet and eliminate your consumption of citrus juices. Keep eliminating beverages one by one to see if you notice any improvements.

Another method to determine which beverage is the culprit is to eliminate all possible offenders for a prescribed amount of time. If your symptoms improve, consider gradually reintroducing the various drinks one at a time. For instance, add a small glass of orange juice to your breakfast and see if your symptoms return. If they do, eliminate the orange juice and try reintroducing sodas to your diet. You may find that more than one beverage is to blame for your symptoms.

In some cases, you may not need to completely eliminate troublesome beverages; simply restricting the amount you drink may be adequate to provide some relief. For example, if you drink ten cups of coffee a day, you may notice improvement by scaling back to one single cup per day.

Reducing your intake of alcohol can be beneficial in more ways than one. As mentioned previously, alcohol not only increases urine production, too much alcohol can also diminish your ability to recognize the need to urinate and impair your ability to react to urges in time. By cutting back on alcoholic beverages, you may notice an improvement in your bladder control.

■ Can I improve my condition by changing how much I drink throughout the day?

In some cases, making an adjustment in the amount of fluids you consume may make a difference in your symptoms. Common guidelines suggest drinking six to eight eight-ounce glasses of fluids daily. However, you may require more or less than this depending on your activity level, your geographic region, and even the daily temperature. If you are consuming more liquids than you need throughout the day, you may need to reduce your intake. However, before you cut back on your beverages, it's a good idea to ask your doctor approximately how much you should be drinking each day.

Remember that limiting your consumption of fluids too much may prevent you from maintaining proper hydration, and dehydration can actually make your symptoms worse. Without enough fluids, your urine will become more concentrated, which can irritate the bladder and trigger symptoms of urgency and urinary leakage. Therefore, if you have been severely restricting your fluid intake in an effort to avoid accidents, your doctor may actually advise you to increase the amount of beverages you consume.

If you tend to experience urinary leakage at night while you sleep, or you have to get up to use the bathroom several times a night, you may want to limit the amount of fluid you drink in the evening. In this case, you can simply drink most of your daily fluids during the morning and afternoon hours rather than during the evening hours. This may help curtail your nighttime incontinence.

■ Can dietary changes alleviate symptoms of incontinence?

In some instances, changes in your diet may improve your symptoms. As mentioned earlier, spicy foods, acidic foods, pickled foods, artificial sweeteners, and many other foods can irritate the bladder, causing symptoms of urgency or episodes of urinary leakage. Avoiding foods that irritate your bladder can be helpful in reducing incontinence. In many cases, simply reducing your consumption of these foods can be enough to bring about an improvement in your symptoms.

Review the list of foods that act as bladder irritants in chapter 2 to see if there are any foods on the list that you eat on a regular basis. If so, consider cutting down on your consumption of those items. Your doctor may recommend that you eliminate all offending foods from your diet for a period of time or may suggest that you try cutting down on foods one at a time. If you don't notice any positive changes in your symptoms after restricting your consumption for the prescribed time period, your doctor may advise you to gradually add certain foods back to your diet. In many cases, you may find that several different foods bring on your symptoms. In other instances, you may discover that a single food is to blame.

Eliminating certain foods from your diet may not be easy. Giving up foods you enjoy can be difficult. In addition, you may not realize that common offenders like artificial sweeteners may be used in a variety of packaged foods. It's a good idea to start looking at nutrition labels carefully to avoid any foods that bring on your symptoms.

In addition, if you have a tendency to be constipated, you may need to make some changes to your diet. Because constipation and stool impaction can contribute to urinary leakage, you should adopt a healthful diet that promotes good bowel function. One of the best ways to do this is to add fiber to your diet. When you increase your fiber intake, you may also need to add more fluids to your diet.

Getting more fiber in your diet is easy—simply add high-fiber foods, such as whole grains, brown rice, legumes, fruits, and vegetables. You can also take a fiber supplement to increase your daily intake. Note that some high-fiber fruits and vegetables may also be bladder irritants, so choose accordingly. Here is a brief list of high-fiber foods that are not bladder irritants:

- Whole-wheat bread
- Brown rice
- Oatmeal
- Broccoli
- Green peas
- Corn
- Spinach

- Squash
- Kidney beans
- Pinto beans
- Boysenberries
- Blackberries
- Pears
- Raspberries

■ Is it beneficial to lose weight if I'm overweight?

If you're overweight, and especially if you're obese, losing weight can be one of the best ways to reduce the severity of your symptoms. As mentioned earlier, extra weight in the abdomen increases the amount of pressure on the bladder and weakens the muscles of the pelvic floor. These are two common contributors to incontinence.

Losing weight reduces the amount of pressure on your bladder, something that can reduce or even eliminate your symptoms. You may be pleasantly surprised to discover that you don't need to lose large amounts of weight to see positive results. In fact, shedding less than ten pounds may be enough to diminish urinary leakage in some cases.

One particular medical study showed that losing as little as 5 to 10 percent of your body weight is linked to a reduction in episodes of urinary incontinence. That means if you weigh 160 pounds, losing anywhere from 8 to 16 pounds may be all it takes to see an improvement. Of course, maintaining that weight loss is essential to keeping urinary incontinence symptoms at a diminished level. If you regain the weight you lost, your symptoms may return at their previous level of severity.

■ If I quit smoking, will that be helpful?

Smoking affects bladder control in a number of ways, which is why it may be beneficial for you to quit smoking. Even if you have been smoking for many years, and even if you're a heavy smoker, quitting can reverse many of the damages that lead to urinary incontinence.

For instance, smoking reduces production of the hormone estrogen, causing a thinning of the tissues of the pelvic floor and a weakening of the pelvic floor muscles. When you stop smoking cigarettes, the tissues of your pelvic floor may be revitalized. Thinning of the tissues can be reversed, and elasticity that had been lost may return. This means your pelvic floor muscles may regain the ability to contract appropriately to avoid urinary leakage.

In addition, cigarette smoke contains bladder irritants, which can cause symptoms of urgency and leakage. Quitting smoking will eliminate those bladder irritants from your body. Without those irritants, your bladder and urethra may return to functioning normally rather than contracting and opening at inappropriate times. In many instances, symptoms of urgency and urinary leakage may diminish or disappear completely.

Heavy smokers often acquire a chronic cough. As explained previously, a smoker's cough can place additional pressure on the bladder and urethra, leading to episodes of stress incontinence and pelvic organ prolapse. When you stop smoking, the cough may be reduced, or it may go away entirely. This will reduce or eliminate the extra pressure on the urinary tract, resulting in fewer episodes of urinary leakage. It may also reduce your chances of developing pelvic organ prolapse. However, if you already have pelvic organ prolapse, quitting smoking will not reverse this condition.

Smoking also raises your risk of developing bladder cancer or cancer of the urethral lining, both of which can cause urinary incontinence. Kicking the habit will lower your risk for these cancers. Unfortunately, quitting smoking will not eliminate cancer if you already have it.

■ If medication I'm taking is contributing to incontinence, is there anything I can do about it?

As mentioned earlier, many prescription and over-the-counter medications, vitamins, and supplements affect bladder control. Some increase urine production, causing symptoms of frequency and urgency. Some cause the urethra to relax, preventing it from closing tightly enough to keep urine from leaking. Some constrict the urethra, leading to urgency and overflow incontinence. Others irritate the bladder or impair your ability to react quickly enough to urges to urinate. Because so many drugs can cause incontinence, it is important to inform your physician about every type of medication you are taking. He or she can help you determine if it would be beneficial for you to change any of your medications.

If you're taking any over-the-counter medications, vitamins, or supplements that are known to cause symptoms of incontinence, consider stopping them for a while. If your symptoms improve, you may want to stop taking them permanently. Or, if it's something you would like to continue taking, perhaps restart it on a gradual basis. If your symptoms return, check with your local pharmacist or your doctor to see if a different brand may work better for you.

In some cases, you may be taking a prescription medicine that is contributing to your incontinence. In this instance, do not simply stop taking the medication. Discuss it with your doctor first because it may be harmful to abruptly discontinue certain medications. Your doctor may suggest you try a different dosage of the same medication, a different brand of the same type of medication, or a different class of drug. Other brands or classes of drugs may provide the same benefits without causing any bladder side effects.

In addition, it's important to realize that various medications may interact in a negative way when taken together. This means that when taken alone, the drugs might not produce any incontinence side effects, but when combined, they bring on symptoms of urgency or urinary leakage. This is why it is critical that you tell your doctor about every medication, vitamin, and supplement you are taking. Your doctor can help you manage your medications to ensure that they are not contributing to incontinence.

Bladder Training

Bladder training involves teaching yourself to delay urination when you feel the need to go. Instead of racing to the bathroom every time you feel the urge, try to hold off, gradually increasing the time you wait. In the beginning, you may want to try waiting for five minutes after you sense the need to urinate. The following week, try increasing the delay to ten minutes. Continue increasing the length of time each week until you are only urinating once every two to four hours.

Delaying urination may be difficult at first, so you may want to begin your bladder training at home where you have access to the bathroom and a change of clothes if necessary. In public places, you may have to wait in line to use the bathroom so factor that into your timed delays. There are also a few techniques you can use to help you wait out the delay. For instance, you can try taking slow, deep breaths until the urge passes. Crossing your legs tightly or distracting yourself with an activity may also help you make it through the delay.

As part of your bladder training, your doctor may instruct you to practice something called double voiding. This means that after you urinate, you wait a few minutes and then try to go again. Double voiding can help train you to empty your bladder more completely.

Bladder training is commonly recommended to help control urge and overflow incontinence. By learning to control the urges and to empty your bladder more completely, you may be able to reduce the likelihood of an accident.

■ What is timed voiding?

Another type of bladder training is timed voiding. With this technique, you go to the bathroom at set intervals whether you feel the urge to go or not. When you first begin timed voiding, you may need to urinate once every hour or even once every half hour. Let's use once an hour as an example. As it becomes easier for you to wait one hour between bathroom breaks, increase the amount of time by fifteen minutes. This means that you will now schedule yourself to urinate once every hour and fifteen minutes. Try to increase the time interval by about fifteen minutes each week until you are going once every two to four hours.

As you increase the amount of time between your trips to the bathroom, you may need to use some of the techniques mentioned previously to avoid episodes of urinary leakage. Breathing deeply and distracting yourself with activities can be beneficial in waiting out the additional minutes. If you find that you are having trouble increasing your intervals one week, simply stay at the previous week's schedule and try again the following week.

■ How does a voiding diary help with the bladder training process?

Keeping a voiding diary that records fluid intake, output, and leakage episodes can be very helpful in bladder training. If you're on a timed voiding schedule, it can help ensure that you remain on your schedule. The simple act of writing down the time of each bathroom break can help you stay on track. If you don't record each trip to the bathroom, you may find yourself wondering whether or not you went.

Your voiding diary is also a good source for monitoring your progress. You may find that after a few weeks, you're urinating with less frequency. In some cases, you may be feeling less of a sense of urgency when you need to go, or you may be having fewer episodes of urinary leakage. Seeing positive improvement can help keep you motivated to continue your bladder training.

A voiding diary can also alert you to urinary trends. For instance, you may notice that you tend to feel more urgency or have leakage an hour after you drink a cup of coffee and a glass of orange juice and eat a bowl of cereal with milk for breakfast. In this instance, the coffee and orange juice may be irritating your bladder or you may simply be ingesting too many liquids at once. You may discover that eliminating the bladder-irritating beverages or spreading out your beverages throughout the morning rather than drinking them all at once reduces your symptoms.

■ How long does it take to see improvement from bladder training?

In some cases, you may begin to see positive results from bladder training in as little as three to six weeks. Other times, signs of improvement may take closer to two or three months. If after three months you aren't seeing any results, you should discuss it with your doctor. In some cases, you may require other types of therapy.

Note that even if you do notice a decrease in your overall symptoms, you may have occasional setbacks. Don't be discouraged. This is normal. As long as you're seeing generally positive results, you should continue with the program. In fact, you need to remember that bladder training requires an ongoing commitment. Even if you have reached your goal of urinating only once every two to four hours and you've got leakage under control, you need to continue practicing these urinary habits. If you resort back to your old habits, your symptoms may return.

Exercises

Exercises that target the muscles of the pelvic floor may improve or even eliminate your symptoms in some cases. Pelvic floor exercises (PFE) are commonly called *Kegel exercises.* They are named after Dr. Arnold Kegel, a Los Angeles gynecologist who, in the late 1940s, was the first to promote the idea of pelvic floor exercises to treat incontinence.

Just as jogging strengthens your legs and lifting weights tones your arms, exercising can strengthen the pelvic floor muscles. Remember, your pelvic floor muscles play an important role in bladder control—they open and close the urethra, and they provide support for the bladder to keep it in its proper position within the pelvis. As explained previously, weakened pelvic floor muscles are linked to stress and urge incontinence.

Strengthening these muscles with exercise can improve your ability to control your bladder. Pelvic floor exercises are commonly recommended as a first line of treatment option for incontinence and are especially effective in treating stress incontinence. They may also reduce symptoms associated with urge incontinence.

■ How are Kegel exercises performed and how often should I do them?

To gain the maximum benefits of Kegel exercises, you need to make sure you perform them correctly. Your doctor can inform you how to perform these exercises and may have a diagram or handout that you can take home with you. Even so, perfecting Kegel exercises may take some practice.

Finding the Pelvic Floor Muscles

The first step in performing Kegel exercises is finding the right muscles in your pelvic floor. There are several methods you can use to identify these muscles.

■ While urinating, try to stop the flow of urine. The muscles you engage to halt the flow are the same pelvic floor muscles you'll be using when you perform Kegel exercises. This method should be used only as a way to identify your pelvic floor muscles because routinely stopping the flow of urine can cause urinary infections and can actually weaken the pelvic muscles.

■ Tighten your rectum as if you were trying to avoid passing gas or as if you were trying to pinch off a stool. You should feel a pulling or closing sensation in your genital area as you do this.

■ Another method is to insert one of your fingers into your vagina and try to squeeze it with the surrounding muscles. You should be able to feel your pelvic floor muscles tighten and shift upward. When you relax your muscles, you should notice the pelvic floor move downward.

As you try to identify your pelvic floor muscles, make sure you aren't using the muscles in your legs, buttocks, or abdomen. The key to performing the exercises correctly is isolating the pelvic floor muscles. If you aren't sure if you've located the right muscles, don't hesitate to ask your doctor for help in identifying them.

Pelvic Floor Exercise Contractions

There are two types of contractions involved in performing pelvic floor exercises: the long hold and the quick flick.

■ *Long hold:* The long hold is an endurance contraction that improves support for your pelvic organs. To perform a long hold, slowly tighten your pelvic floor muscles and hold the contraction for up to ten seconds. Then relax the muscles for the same number of seconds. Repeat the squeezing five to ten times with a rest between each hold. Each week, increase the amount of time you hold the contraction. As your strength improves, you should be able to tighten your muscles for ten seconds or longer. As the length of the hold increases, be sure to increase the amount of rest time to match the squeeze time. For instance, if you can squeeze your pelvic floor muscles for eight seconds, then rest for eight seconds in between each squeeze. If you can hold for ten seconds, rest for ten seconds.

■ *Quick flick:* These are a series of fast, strong contractions lasting only a couple of seconds each. These exercises increase your ability to prevent leakage when you cough, sneeze, or strain. To perform the quick flick, simply tighten the pelvic floor muscles as hard as you can and then relax them completely. Begin with a series of five to ten squeezes and releases. Each week, gradually increase the number of quick flicks you perform.

When to Perform Pelvic Floor Exercises

Many physical therapists who specialize in pelvic floor training recommend performing pelvic floor exercises at least five times a day. For instance, you could do five to ten quick flicks and five to ten long holds while you are still in bed in the morning, at lunchtime, in the afternoon, at dinnertime, and in bed at night. Although doing the exercises five times a day is a common approach, you may want to ask your doctor to help you create an individualized pelvic floor exercise routine. Your doctor's recommendations on the number of repetitions you should perform and the number of times you should do them each day may differ slightly from the recommendations in this book.

In addition to doing Kegel exercises on a routine basis, it is also a good idea to perform these exercises when you are experiencing symptoms of urgency, when you are likely to leak urine, or when you actually are leaking urine. For instance, if you are feeling a sense of urgency, contracting and holding your pelvic floor muscles may help you hold your urine until you can get to a bathroom. If you have stress incontinence, performing a contraction when you are about to cough or sneeze may prevent leakage. If you are leaking urine on your way to the bathroom, contracting your pelvic muscles may stop the leaking.

Where to Perform Pelvic Floor Exercises

You can perform Kegel exercises anywhere at anytime. You can do them while driving, while sitting at your desk at work, or while you're lying in bed. You can even do them in a crowded room, and the people around you won't know it. Kegel exercises can be performed in a lying, sitting, or standing position. In the beginning, it may be easier to perform them lying down. As the strength of your pelvic floor muscles increases, you may progress to doing your exercises sitting or standing.

Pelvic Floor Exercise Tips

■ Be sure to empty your bladder before performing either long hold or quick flick contractions. Doing

Kegel exercises with a full bladder can lead to urinary tract infections and other problems.

- If you have stress incontinence, try making a voluntary cough while doing your Kegel exercises. This way, when you have an involuntary cough, you will automatically do a contraction.

- Breathe normally while performing Kegel exercises.

- Don't use the muscles of your legs, abdomen, or buttocks while contracting your pelvic floor muscles. Isolating the muscles of the pelvic floor will provide maximum results.

- **Is there any way to know if I am performing the exercises correctly?**

If you are having trouble feeling your pelvic floor muscles, a technique called biofeedback may be recommended. Biofeedback is a special monitoring system that lets you know when you are contracting and relaxing the right muscles.

Biofeedback devices typically include a small sensor that is inserted into the vagina, a small electronic unit with a built-in display, and electrodes that adhere to the lower abdomen, thighs, and buttocks. With some devices, electrodes may be used in the pelvic area instead of a sensor. With the sensor probe and electrodes in place, you contract your pelvic floor muscles and the electronic display uses lights and beeps to signal whether or not you are contracting the proper muscles. The electrodes detect if you are contracting the muscles in your legs, abdomen, or buttocks rather than isolating the pelvic floor muscles.

In addition to letting you know if you are contracting the right muscles, many biofeedback devices measure the strength of your pelvic floor contractions. This allows you to note any improvement in your muscle tone over time. Seeing your progress can be a great motivator and may encourage you to keep up with your pelvic floor exercise program.

Initially, biofeedback is typically performed under the supervision of a physical therapist or nurse. If your doctor recommends biofeedback for you, a referral to a physical therapist or nurse can be provided. Once you've gone through a few sessions and understand how biofeedback works, you may want to purchase a small unit for home use. You don't need a prescription for most biofeedback devices, and you can pick them up at any drugstore or medical supply store. Costs range from ten dollars to several hundred dollars and may be covered by your insurance.

Studies show that using a biofeedback device can be helpful in relieving your incontinence symptoms. In one study of women under the age of seventy-five using biofeedback, significant improvement was noted in 40 to 50 percent of the women. About 10 to 25 percent of the women reported that their symptoms disappeared completely.

■ What if my pelvic floor muscles are too weak for me to be able to perform the exercises correctly?

If your pelvic floor muscles have become so weakened that you are not able to perform Kegel exercises correctly, don't be discouraged. A technique called electrical stimulation may help you achieve the benefits of pelvic floor exercises. Sometimes referred to as E-stim, this technique provides the controlled delivery of small amounts of electrical stimulation to the muscles of the pelvic floor. Delivered in small pulses, the electrical stimulation causes your muscles to contract and relax in the same way as if you were contracting the muscles yourself.

If your doctor recommends electrical stimulation, the procedure may be performed in your doctor's office, in a physical therapist's office, or in your own home using a small device. Your doctor may advise you to have the procedure in a medical professional's office at first so you understand how it works prior to your purchasing a device for home use.

Whether you are using a portable home device or you are having electrical stimulation in a doctor's office, the procedure is performed in the same way. A small probe similar to a tampon is inserted into the vagina or the rectum. The probe is connected by a wire to a device that controls the delivery of the electrical stimulation. The amount of electrical stimulation can be increased or decreased to achieve the desired results. In some cases, electrical stimulation may be perceived as painful. In most cases, you should be able to adjust the level of stimulation to contract the muscles without feeling any pain.

Obtaining the maximum benefits from electrical stimulation takes time. A typical regimen may include two fifteen-minute treatment sessions twice a day for at least three months. Although this treatment option takes time, it has been reported that up to 48 percent of women trying the technique see improvement, with some of them experiencing a complete cure of their symptoms. Take note that some insurance companies do not cover electrical stimulation for the treatment of incontinence.

In some instances, a special chair may be used to deliver electrical stimulation. The chair has an electromagnet under the seat that delivers electrical pulses to the muscles of the pelvic area. You simply sit in the chair fully clothed, and the pulses cause your pelvic floor muscles to contract and relax. A typical regimen may require you to sit in the chair for about twenty minutes two times a week for at least two months.

Chair therapy may sound appealing because it requires no effort other than a time commitment on your part. However, you should realize that your symptoms may return once you stop chair therapy, or you may require ongoing follow-ups to maintain positive results. In addition, the specialized chairs are not widely available and only a few urologists, gynecologists, and urogynecologists have them in their offices.

■ How long does it usually take to see results from pelvic floor therapy?

In most cases, it can take three to six months to see long-term results from pelvic floor exercises. However, you may begin to see some improvement within eight to twelve weeks. Because it can take months to notice a decrease in your symptoms, you may find it difficult to stick with the program. If you don't see results right away, don't get discouraged. Pelvic floor therapy simply takes time and patience.

■ **How can I stay motivated to continue a pelvic floor exercise program?**

Keeping a diary of your pelvic floor exercises may help you stay on track. Make it a practice to record the number of long hold and quick flick contractions you can do each time, along with the length of time you can hold a long contraction. This way, you may begin to see progress in the strength of your pelvic floor even if you aren't managing to stay dry yet. The sense of achievement you feel may encourage you to continue your exercises until you begin to see a decrease your symptoms.

■ **Is there anything I can do to make Kegel exercises work faster?**

Specially designed vaginal weights can be used to help you identify the muscles of the pelvic floor and may accelerate your pelvic floor therapy. Vaginal weights range from less than an ounce to about half a pound and may be shaped like lozenges or barbells. Most vaginal weights have a string attached for easy removal from the vagina.

Using vaginal weights is simple. You insert the weight into your vagina and contract your pelvic floor muscles in order to hold it in place. You should be able to sense your muscles squeezing around the weight, which lets you know that you are using the correct pelvic floor muscles. It is recommended to hold the weight within the vagina for up to fifteen minutes at a time, two times a day for at least three months.

When you begin a pelvic floor therapy program using vaginal weights, start with the lowest weight and gradually work up to heavier weights. In the beginning, you may need to lie down while you hold the weight in place. As your muscles become stronger, try standing up and walking around with the weight inserted. When you are easily able to walk around with the insert in place for at least fifteen minutes, you should try jogging in place or coughing. If you arc ablc to do so without leaking urine, you've made real progress.

Once you have strengthened your pelvic floor muscles with vaginal weights, your symptoms of urgency and stress incontinence may decrease or disappear entirely. Studies show that up to 38 percent of women who follow a pelvic floor therapy regimen using vaginal weights for at least three months will experience a cure of stress incontinence. Studies report more-modest improvements in symptoms associated with urge incontinence.

Even if you do notice improvement, however, it doesn't mean that you can stop the program. Pelvic floor therapy requires an ongoing commitment, and you may need to continue using your vaginal weights from time to time to maintain the positive results you have achieved.

■ **Is it more effective to combine lifestyle changes with bladder training and pelvic floor exercises?**

In most cases, you are more likely to reduce symptoms of incontinence when you combine behavior therapies. For instance, if you lose weight, quit smoking, practice bladder training, and do pelvic floor exercises, you have a much better chance of seeing improvement than if you only quit smoking or only practice bladder training. Consult with your doctor to determine what combination of behavior modifications is most likely to improve your situation.

■ **What if I don't see any improvement after three months of lifestyle changes and Kegel exercises?**

If after three months you still aren't noticing any improvement, consult with your doctor. You may discover that you haven't been doing your pelvic floor exercises correctly, or you may require other types of treatment.

Chapter 5

Treating Incontinence with Medication

In some instances, medication may be recommended to help you control incontinence. In fact, for a number of reasons, drug therapy is being used more commonly now to treat more drugs are available to treat the condition than ever before. The wider variety of medications on the market means that physicians are better able to find a drug that fits your particular needs. Thanks to ads for incontinence drugs that are now appearing on television and in magazines, there is a growing awareness of medication as a treatment option for this problem. Due to this increased awareness, women may be more likely to ask their doctors about medication to treat their symptoms.

It is important to understand that many of the drugs advertised on TV are designed to treat one specific type of urinary problem—usually overactive bladder. If you have a different type of incontinence, these drugs may not be right for you. Finding the appropriate medication for you is highly individual and depends on the type of incontinence you have. Incontinence medication may be prescribed alone, but it is often recommended in conjunction with conservative therapy, such as pelvic floor exercises, bladder training, and lifestyle changes. In many cases, combining medication with behavior modifications can enhance their effectiveness.

■ What are the various types of medications available to treat incontinence?

Medications approved by the Food and Drug Administration (FDA) to treat incontinence come in a variety of forms, including oral drugs, topical skin patches, and topical creams. In addition, some drugs that are designed to treat problems other than incontinence appear to improve incontinence symptoms. Using such medications is referred to as *off-label usage*. This means the drugs are being used to treat a condition other than what they were originally intended to treat.

Incontinence drugs are gaining popularity in part thanks to more-convenient dosing. In the past, many medications required you to take pills two or three times a day. Now, several oral drugs require only a single pill a day. Many of the drugs have also been refined, making them more effective at improving symptoms. Thanks to this added convenience and efficacy, doctors are more likely to prescribe medication either as a long-term solution or as a short-term fix until conservative therapy starts showing positive results.

Lower costs are also contributing to the growing use of incontinence medications. Less-expensive generic versions of some of the drugs have become available, making them more affordable. In addition, many health care plans cover some or all of the costs associated with these drugs.

■ Can all types of incontinence be treated with medication?

Some types of incontinence are more successfully treated with medication than others. For example, medications designed to treat overactive bladder and urge incontinence have proven to be the most effective. Medical studies report that 83 percent of women taking incontinence medication experience a reduction in urge incontinence, with up to 43 percent of patients experiencing complete elimination of symptoms.

Medications that treat overflow incontinence have a lower rate of success in reducing symptoms. As for stress incontinence, there are currently no medications available that have been approved by the FDA. Still, some improvement in stress incontinence symptoms has been noted using off-label drugs. In addition to the medications currently available, medical professionals continue to test new drugs in an effort to help find relief for patients with urinary incontinence.

■ How do medications to treat incontinence work?

Medications used to treat incontinence affect the bladder in a variety of ways to reduce symptoms. For instance, some drugs relax the bladder and reduce the bladder contractions that lead to involuntary urine loss. Some drugs improve bladder muscle tone or strengthen the muscles surrounding the urethra so it can close more effectively to reduce the risk of leakage. Other medications aim to improve the condition of the tissues of the pelvic floor, thereby allowing them to contract and expand as needed for normal urination and reducing the risk of urgency and leakage.

■ When are medications prescribed?

Depending on your diagnosis, medication may be prescribed following an initial evaluation. In many cases, medication is recommended in conjunction with conservative therapy, such as weight loss, smoking cessation, pelvic floor therapy, and lifestyle changes. Sometimes, the medication is used to provide temporary relief from your symptoms until you begin to see results from conservative therapy. In this case, if and when conservative therapy results in improvement, you may be able to decrease your medication or stop taking it entirely.

If you are looking for a quick fix for incontinence, medication may offer some relief. However, it may be in your best interest to combine medication with conservative therapy, which may eventually provide you with long-lasting improvement. In some cases, medication may be prescribed as an interim fix while you wait for a more long-term solution for incontinence, such as surgery. In this situation, drugs may minimize symptoms until a permanent repair is achieved. There are also instances where medication may be necessary as a long-term solution.

■ Do medications provide immediate relief from symptoms?

With the right medication in the proper dosage, symptoms typically improve in about two weeks. In some cases, however, it may take longer. Aside from how long it takes the medication to start working, your doctor may also have to adjust the dosage to achieve the best results. Your physician may begin with a low dosage of a mild drug. If that doesn't improve your situation, he or she may recommend a higher dosage of the same drug or a stronger medication. Minor adjustments may continue to be required until you start seeing improvement.

■ Which medications are currently available to treat urge incontinence and overactive bladder?

There is a wide variety of medications currently available to treat urge incontinence and overactive bladder. In fact, there are more medications available to treat these conditions than any other type of incontinence. Most of the drugs are pills that you take orally, but drugs are also available in a skin patch, in topical creams, and in injections. Drugs your physician may recommend include the following.

Anticholinergics

These drugs work by blocking the nerve impulses to the bladder that cause abnormal contractions and contribute to leakage. Blocking the nerve impulses relaxes the bladder, decreasing involuntary bladder spasms, reducing the strength of these contractions, and increasing the amount of urine your bladder can hold. All of this adds up to fewer episodes of urgency, frequency, and leakage.

Anticholinergic medications that have been approved by the FDA to treat overactive bladder and urge incontinence include oxybutynin (Ditropan, Ditropan XL, Oxytrol), tolterodine (Detrol, Detrol LA), solifenacin (VESIcare), darifenacin (Enablex), and trospium (Sanctura). Ditropan has been used for decades and was the first incontinence drug approved by the FDA in 1975. An extended-release version of the drug, Ditropan XL, earned approval in 1998. The FDA approved Detrol in 1998 and Detrol LA, an extended-release pill, in 2000. Oxytrol was approved in 2003. VESIcare, Enablex, and Sanctura—all extended-release pills—each earned FDA approval in 2004.

All of these drugs come in the form of an oral pill except Oxytrol, which is sold as a skin patch. Some of the oral drugs require you to take pills two or three times a day. The extended-release forms require only one pill a day.

In many cases, if your doctor recommends oxybutynin, you will have a choice of taking an oral drug or using a skin patch. The Oxytrol skin patch delivers oxybutynin, the same medication found in the oral drug Ditropan, through the skin into the bloodstream. It is a thin, clear, flexible patch that is applied to the hip, abdomen, or buttock. The patch continuously delivers the oxybutynin for up to four days. Typically, two patches are required each week. To make it easier to remember when to change your patch, always change it on the same two days of the week.

If you have a spinal cord injury, your physician may recommend that you use Ditropan in the bladder as a wash. This is performed by crushing up your pills and inserting them into the bladder directly using a catheter.

The drug your physician recommends often depends on the severity of your symptoms. For instance, Detrol or Detrol LA may be recommended for mild symptoms, Enablex or VESIcare may be better suited for moderate symptoms, and Sanctura, Ditropan, or Ditropan XL may be the drug of choice for severe cases.

Although these drugs may provide relief for your symptoms of urgency and incontinence, remember that they are associated with a number of side effects. Dry mouth is the most common side effect and can be severe in some people. If you experience dry mouth, your first inclination may be to consume more fluids. But increasing your fluid intake may actually increase symptoms of urgency, frequency, and leakage, nullifying the beneficial effects of the medication.

Other side effects include dry eye, constipation, headache, abdominal pain, a worsening of acid reflux, hypertension, drowsiness, urinary retention, blurred vision, and mental confusion. Because of these last two side effects, these drugs may not be recommended if you have glaucoma, Alzheimer's disease, or dementia. In some cases, the side effects associated with drugs for overactive bladder and urge incontinence may be so troublesome that you may feel the downside outweighs the benefits. Dry mouth is the side effect most often cited for stopping the medication.

Studies show that the Oxytrol skin patch typically poses less risk for these side effects. However, it may cause skin irritations. You can help avoid skin irritations by placing each new patch in a different area from the previous patch. For instance, you may want to place your first patch of the week on one side of your body and the second patch of the week on the opposite side.

There is no way of knowing beforehand if you will experience side effects from any of these drugs. If you do experience some discomfort, it is important to tell your doctor. Your physician may recommend a different dosage of the same drug to minimize side effects or may prescribe a different drug to see if you tolerate it better.

Most anticholinergic medications are available in brand name only, which can be expensive. In fact, only one of these drugs, oxybutynin, is currently available in an inexpensive generic form. In general, the extended-release pills that are taken once a day cost more than the pills that must be taken two to three times a day. Depending on your insurance provider, some or all of the costs of generic or brand-name anticholinergics may be covered.

Medications for Urge Incontinence and Overactive Bladder

Generic Name	Brand Name	Usage
Oxybutynin	Ditropan	2–3 times a day
	Ditropan XL	Once a day
	Oxytrol (skin patch)	2 times a week
Tolterodine	Detrol	2 times a day
	Detrol LA	Once a day
Solifenacin	VESIcare	Once a day
Darifenacin	Enablex	Once a day
Trospium	Sanctura	2 times a day

Alpha-adrenergic Inhibitors

Also known as alpha-adrenergic blockers, these drugs were originally created to treat high blood pressure. They have also been used to treat men with an enlarged prostate. With off-label usage, alpha-adrenergic inhibitors have shown positive results in treating women with overactive bladder and overflow incontinence. By relaxing the bladder neck and urethra, these drugs improve your ability to empty your bladder more completely, leaving you with less residual urine in your bladder. They may also decrease symptoms of urgency and frequency.

Alpha-adrenergic inhibitors are taken orally in pill form. Currently, there are four alpha-adrenergic blockers that may be prescribed, including tamsulosin (Flomax), doxazosin (Cardura), terazosin (Hytrin), and alfuzosin (Uroxatral). Each of these drugs is available as an extended-release pill, which means you only need to take them once a day.

Side effects of alpha-adrenergic inhibitors include runny nose, dizziness, low blood pressure, fatigue, and vertigo. In some cases, these drugs may actually increase episodes of incontinence. This can occur if there is too much relaxation of the bladder neck and urethra so that they no longer close tightly enough to prevent leakage. Currently, only terazosin and doxazosin are available in a less-expensive generic form. More recently, a generic form of tamsulosin was recently approved by the FDA. Alfuzosin is only available as Uroxatral. Alpha-adrenergic inhibitors are covered by most insurance plans. Depending on your particular plan, some or all of the costs of these medications may be covered.

Medications for Overactive Bladder and Overflow Incontinence

Generic Name	Brand Name	Usage
Tamsulosin	Flomax	Once a day
Doxazosin	Cardura	Once a day
Terazosin	Hytrin	Once a day
Alfuzocin	Uroxatral	Once a day

Imipramine (Tofranil, Tofranil-PM)

Tofranil is the brand name for the generic drug imipramine, which is approved by the FDA as an antidepressant. With off-label usage, imipramine has also been found to alleviate symptoms of mixed incontinence, overactive bladder, urgency, urge incontinence, and stress incontinence.

Imipramine provides benefits associated with both anticholinergics and alpha-adrenergic inhibitors. Its anticholinergic effect decreases bladder contractions, and its alpha-adrenergic blocker effect increases the urethra's ability to close tightly. The dual-action benefits can lead to fewer episodes of leakage, urgency, and frequency.

Like anticholinergics, imipramine can cause side effects, such as dry mouth, constipation, and blurry vision. It may also trigger the fatigue and dizziness associated with alpha-adrenergic inhibitors. In addition, the drug can cause serious side effects affecting the cardiovascular system, including low blood pressure, rapid heartbeat, and irregular heartbeat. In some cases, the drug may make it more difficult for you to urinate due to the decreased bladder contractions and increased urethra closure.

Estrogen (Premarin Vaginal Cream, Estring, Vagifem)

If you are postmenopausal, estrogen may be recommended to treat the symptoms of overactive bladder, urge incontinence, stress incontinence, or mixed incontinence. Following menopause, estrogen production decreases, sometimes reducing the strength and flexibility of the supportive tissues of the pelvic floor.

Scientific theories suggest that estrogen therapy may reverse the weakening of these tissues and, in turn, improve bladder control. In addition, there is evidence that estrogen therapy decreases postmenopausal symptoms of frequency and urgency and decreases the risk of recurrent urinary tract infections, a potential cause of incontinence. However, some medical studies have shown little proof that estrogen therapy can improve urinary incontinence.

Estrogen therapy is available in pill form and as a topical application. Oral drugs do not appear to produce the same beneficial effects as topical estrogen, and they may pose serious health risks, including increased risk for heart attacks, strokes, breast cancer, blood clots, and dementia. For these reasons, topical estrogen is typically recommended for symptoms of urge incontinence, stress incontinence, or overactive bladder.

Topical estrogen is available in a variety of forms, including creams, vaginal rings, and tablets. These drugs do not appear to carry the same risks as oral estrogen. That's because estrogen that is applied directly to the vaginal area is less likely to be absorbed into the bloodstream. However, be aware that all estrogens increase the chances of developing cancer in the lining of the uterus. If you notice any unusual vaginal bleeding while using a topical estrogen product, contact your doctor. Estrogen cream (Premarin Vaginal Cream) is inserted into the vagina using an applicator and releases the drug into the vagina. Dosages and recommendations differ, but a typical treatment plan may begin with approximately three weeks of daily usage and continue with twice-weekly usage. With a vaginal estrogen cream, you may experience positive results within three weeks. Side effects include vaginal pain, breast pain, vaginitis, and itching.

Topical Estrogen Therapy

Generic Name	Brand Name	Usage
Conjugated estrogens vaginal cream	Premarin Vaginal Cream	Once daily or twice weekly
Estradiol vaginal ring	Estring	Once every three months
Estradiol vaginal tablets	Vagifem	Once daily or twice weekly

The estradiol vaginal ring (Estring) continuously delivers estrogen into the vagina. Made of pliable elastomer (rubber), the ring is slightly larger in diameter than a quarter. The ring is inserted high into the vagina and remains in place for three months at a time. You simply use your finger to insert and remove the ring. Side effects of the vaginal estrogen ring include abdominal pain, back pain, nausea, headaches, vaginal discharge, and vaginal infection.

Estradiol vaginal tablets (Vagifem), which may also be called estrogen suppositories, are inserted into the vagina using an applicator. They dissolve gradually, releasing estrogen directly to the vaginal tissues. A typical treatment plan involves inserting one estrogen tablet daily for two weeks and then inserting one tablet twice a week thereafter. You may begin to see improvement after as little as two weeks.

■ Are any drugs recommended to treat stress incontinence?

Currently, no drugs have been approved by the FDA to treat stress incontinence. However, off-label usage of a number of medications may be recommended to alleviate symptoms. These drugs include alpha-adrenergic stimulants, duloxetine, imipramine, and estrogen.

Alpha-adrenergic Stimulants

Also called alpha-agonists, these medications contain pseudoephedrine and are typically found in dozens of over-the-counter nasal decongestants and diet pills, as well as in some prescription allergy medicines. Common over-the-counter and prescription drugs containing pseudoephedrine include Sudafed, Claritin-D, Clarinex-D, Sinutab, Zyrtec-D, Allegra-D, and Advil Cold & Sinus, among others.

Although they are not approved by the FDA for the treatment of incontinence, these medications have shown some effectiveness in reducing the symptoms associated with stress incontinence. These drugs have the opposite effect of alpha-adrenergic inhibitors. While the inhibitors relax the bladder neck and urethra, the stimulants cause them to close more tightly. This can help prevent urinary leakage when you cough, sneeze, or stand up from a sitting position. However, in many cases, improvement tends to be minimal, which is why alpha-adrenergic stimulants are not frequently recommended.

Alpha-adrenergic stimulants may cause side effects, including insomnia, increased pulse rate, increased blood pressure, headache, and dizziness. They may also increase the risk of heart attack and stroke. In some cases, these drugs can cause too much tightening of the urethra, leading to problems emptying your bladder.

Duloxetine (Cymbalta)

Originally approved by the FDA to treat depression, duloxetine may also be prescribed to treat stress incontinence with off-label usage. Sold under the brand name Cymbalta, the drug is believed to increase contraction of the urethral sphincter. Tightening of the urethra can help prevent cough or sneeze.

Duloxetine is generally taken once a day, and may be covered by insurance. Side effects of the drug include nausea, dry mouth, constipation, diarrhea, heartburn, decreased appetite, cough, sweating, insomnia, blurred vision, dizziness, fatigue, runny nose, muscle pain, and changes in sexual desire. Nausea is the most common side effect. Note that higher dosages of the drug tend to increase the risk of side effects.

Imipramine (Tofranil, Tofranil-PM)

As described previously, the antidepressant drug imipramine is sometimes prescribed off-label to treat stress incontinence, overactive bladder, urgency, and urge incontinence. The drug's alpha-adrenergic inhibitor effect increases the ability of the urethra to close tightly enough to prevent episodes of stress incontinence, such as leaking when you cough or sneeze. See the previous section on drugs used to treat urge incontinence and overactive bladder for more information on imipramine.

Estrogen (Premarin Vaginal Cream, Estring, Vagifem)

As explained earlier, estrogen may reduce symptoms of stress incontinence, overactive bladder, urge incontinence, or mixed incontinence. If you are postmenopausal, using an estrogen medication may improve the strength and flexibility of the supportive tissues of the pelvic floor. This may reduce your chances of leaking due to weakened pelvic floor muscles. For more information on various estrogen drugs and their side effects, see the previous section on medications that are recommended for urge incontinence and overactive bladder.

■ Which drugs are likely to be prescribed for overflow incontinence?

Medications that may be prescribed to treat overflow incontinence include cholinergics, Valium, alpha-adrenergic inhibitors, and Botox.

Cholinergics (Urecholine)

Whereas anticholinergics relax the bladder and reduce contractions, cholinergics do just the opposite. These drugs stimulate the sacral nerves that signal the bladder when it is time to urinate. This causes an increase in bladder contractions, which may help you empty your bladder more completely. For this reason, cholinergics may be prescribed to treat overflow incontinence.

Cholinergics include bethanechol chloride, which is sold under the brand name Urecholine. If your doctor prescribes Urecholine, you'll need to take three to four pills a day. This drug is commonly covered by insurance. Urecholine's side effects include abdominal cramps, nausea, belching, urinary urgency, skin flushing/sweating, lowered blood pressure with increased pulse rate, headache, salivation, and bronchial constriction/asthmatic symptoms.

Diazepam (Valium)

Typically prescribed as a muscle relaxant, Valium may also relax the urethral outlet or skeletal sphincter muscle. Because of this, the oral medication is sometimes recommended for off-label usage to treat overflow incontinence. When Valium is prescribed to treat incontinence, it is usually taken once a day.

Valium is available in an inexpensive generic form, and it may be covered by insurance. Side effects associated with the drug include drowsiness, depression, nausea, headache, dry mouth, vivid dreams, decreased sex drive, and changes in behavior. If you have glaucoma, you may be advised not to take Valium.

Alpha-adrenergic Inhibitors

As mentioned earlier, alpha-adrenergic inhibitors have been used off-label to treat overflow incontinence as well as overactive bladder. By relaxing the bladder neck and urethra, these drugs allow you to more effectively empty your bladder. In most cases, this results in a decrease in residual urine in your bladder, which can reduce your episodes of overflow incontinence. Additional information about these drugs can be found in the section on drugs used to treat overactive bladder and urge incontinence.

Botulinum Toxin Type A (Botox)

As described previously, Botox is a muscle relaxant. When injected into the bladder, it may relax the bladder and urethra, which can alleviate symptoms associated with overflow incontinence, urge incontinence, and overactive bladder. See the section on medications that are recommended to treat urge incontinence and overactive bladder for more information on Botox injections.

■ **Are there any drugs that are recommended to treat frequency and nighttime incontinence?**

Desmopressin (Stimate, DDAVP) is a chemical form of an antidiuretic hormone (ADH) that is found naturally in the body. This drug decreases urine production and can reduce symptoms of frequency. Desmopressin is usually prescribed to treat bed-wetting in children, but it may also reduce symptoms of frequency in adults. Once commonly prescribed, antidiuretic medication has proven to be only minimally effective and is no longer recommended as often as it was in the past. This medication is available in both a nasal spray and in an oral pill. Usually, you will have to take desmopressin twice a day, but dosages may vary. Your insurance provider may cover some or all of the costs of a prescription. Side effects from the drug include headache, nausea, salt retention, water

89

retention, ankle swelling, pulmonary edema, shortness of breath, and congestive heart failure.

Medications Used to Treat Incontinence

Generic Name	Brand Names	Type of Incontinence
Anticholinergics		
Oxybutynin	Ditropan	Overactive Bladder
	Ditropan XL	Urge
	Oxytrol	
Tolterodine	Detrol	
	Detrol LA	
Solifenacin	VESIcare	
Darifenacin	Enablex	
Trospium	Sanctura	
Cholinergics		
Bethanechol chloride	Urecholine	Overflow
Alpha-adrenergic Inhibitors		
Tamsulosin	Flomax	Overactive Bladder
Doxazosin	Cardura	Overflow
Terazosin	Hytrin	
Alfuzocin	Uroxatral	
Alpha-adrenergic Stimulants		
Pseudoephedrine	Sudafed, Claritin-D,	Stress
	Clarinex-D, Sinutab,	
	Zyrtec-D, Allegra-D,	
	Advil Cold & Sinus, etc.	
Antidepressants		
Imipramine	Tofranil	Stress
	Tofranil-PM	Urge

Generic Name	Brand Names	Type of Incontinence
continued...		
		Overactive Bladder
		Mixed
Duloxetine	Cymbalta	Stress
Estrogon		
Conjugated estrogens vaginal cream	Premarin Vaginal Cream	Stress
Estradiol vaginal ring	Estring	Urge
Estradiol vaginal tablets	Vagifem	Mixed
		Overactive Bladder
Neurotoxins		
Botulinum toxin type A	Botox	Overactive Bladder
		Urge
		Overflow
Muscle Relaxants		
Diazepam	Valium	Overflow
Antidiuretics		
Desmopressin	Stimate DDAVP	Frequency

Chapter 6

Treating Incontinence with Surgery

A number of surgical procedures are used to treat urinary incontinence. Most are designed to treat stress incontinence, but a growing number of surgical options are proving effective in the treatment of urge incontinence and overactive bladder. Thanks to numerous advances in surgical techniques, many incontinence operations are providing better results than they had previously. In addition, a growing number of minimally invasive procedures are being performed, allowing for a quicker recovery with fewer side effects. When performed by a trained specialist, surgery to treat incontinence may provide long-lasting results and, in some cases, immediate relief from leakage.

■ When is surgery recommended to treat incontinence?

A surgical procedure may be recommended when other treatment methods have failed. For instance, when behavior modifications have proven to be ineffective, you may benefit from an operation. Similarly, if medications have failed to control your incontinence, a surgical procedure may be advised.

In addition, if you simply don't have the time or desire to commit to lifelong behavior modifications, surgery may be recommended as an alternative. Surgery may also be advised if you have an anatomical defect, such as pelvic organ prolapse, which may contribute to incontinence.

■ Are there any reasons why surgery might not be recommended?

Surgery to treat incontinence may not be advisable if you are pregnant or are planning on having children in the future. This is because pregnancy and childbirth may stretch or damage pelvic tissues and may reverse repairs made with surgery. In addition, certain health conditions, such as severe heart problems, uncontrolled high blood pressure, untreated diabetes, or morbid obesity, may indicate that you are not a good candidate for surgery.

■ What types of surgery are available for the treatment of incontinence?

Many surgical procedures aim to provide better support for the urethra and bladder. The goal of other procedures is to relax the bladder or to regulate the nerve signals being sent to the bladder. Your urologist or urogynecologist will determine which procedure is best for you depending on the type of incontinence you have.

■ Do incontinence procedures require anesthesia?

To help keep you pain-free during your surgical procedure, some form of anesthesia is typically required. If you feel somewhat anxious about being "put under," rest assured that improvements in drugs and monitoring techniques have made anesthesia safer today than ever before. To ensure your health and well-being, anesthesia should be administered by a physician anesthesiologist or by a certified registered nurse anesthetist (CRNA).

Types of anesthesia that may be used include local, regional, sedation, and general. The anesthesia used during your surgery is determined by the procedure you are having as well as your surgeon's personal preference. Depending on the type of anesthesia that will be administered, you may be asked to refrain from eating or drinking anything after midnight the night before your procedure.

Local Anesthesia

A local anesthetic numbs a small area of the body to prevent pain in that specific location. When this type of anesthesia is used, you remain awake and alert.

Regional

To block pain in a specific region of the body, regional anesthesia is used. Epidurals (commonly used during childbirth) and spinal blocks are examples of regional anesthesia options that prevent or reduce pain in the lower half of the body.

Sedation

A sedative makes you feel relaxed and drowsy and is used in combination with pain medications to minimize discomfort. With this option, you may remain awake during your procedure but may not remember anything once the operation is complete. Sedation may also be called IV sedation, conscious sedation, twilight sedation, or monitored anesthesia care (MAC).

General

With general anesthesia, you are rendered unconscious, will feel no pain, and will have no memory of your operation. General anesthesia prevents you from breathing on your own, so a breathing tube will be inserted down your windpipe (trachea).

■ What should I do to prepare for surgery?

Depending on the type of procedure you are having, you may need to follow special instructions before your operation. These preoperative guidelines are intended to ensure your safety and to improve your chances of achieving the best possible results. In general, minimally invasive procedures involve few preoperative measures. Major surgical procedures, however, may require more-extensive preoperative preparations. Your preoperative instructions may include the following.

Avoid Blood-thinning Medications

Before your procedure, you may be asked to refrain from taking any medication that may thin the blood and interfere with the blood's ability to clot. Examples include aspirin, anti-inflammatory medications, vitamin E, and blood thinners, such as Coumadin. Typically, these medications should be avoided for seven to ten days prior to your procedure. Some patients who require blood thinners to avoid life-threatening clots to the brain or heart may need to use a form of blood thinner right up until the surgery. Your surgeon and primary care physician will decide when is the safest time to stop such medications.

Follow a Special Diet

A special preoperative diet is often advised to prevent postoperative straining when you have a bowel movement, because straining may damage some of the surgical repairs that have been made. You may be advised to avoid constipating foods, such as white rice, bananas, and chocolate, for one week before your operation. You may also be encouraged to consume high-fiber foods, such as oatmeal, cereal, fruits, and vegetables. Your surgeon's staff should provide you with a list of foods to avoid and foods to consume.

The night before your operation, you may be advised to administer an enema to cleanse your bowel. In addition, you will be instructed not to eat, drink, or chew anything after midnight before your procedure. This is a safety measure intended to keep you from aspirating food particles into your lungs during surgery.

Fill Your Prescriptions

If your doctor gives you prescriptions prior to your procedure, get them filled. Medications that may be prescribed include painkillers and antibiotics. Even if you will not need these medications until after your procedure, it is better to have them on hand. In many cases, you may not feel up to going to the pharmacy after your surgery. In some cases, you will be instructed to rest and will not be allowed to drive following your procedure, so you will need to have the medications on hand.

Arrange for a Caregiver

After moderately invasive and major surgical procedures, you may need some assistance as you recover. In many cases, having someone help you with normal household chores and errands for a few days may be all you need. Following major surgical procedures, you may not be able to drive for a few days to a few weeks and you will not be allowed to lift any heavy objects for several weeks. Arranging for someone to be available to give you a ride or to assist you with any heavy lifting can allow your body to get the rest it needs in order to heal properly.

Arrange for Lab Tests

In some cases, you may be required to visit your primary care physician for routine lab tests prior to your procedure. These tests are required to ensure that you are healthy enough to undergo surgery. Lab tests may include a complete blood count (CBC), urinalysis, and electrocardiogram (EKG).

Procedures to Treat Stress Incontinence

A wide variety of surgical options are available to treat stress incontinence. The surgical procedure that is best for you depends on the type of stress incontinence you have. The two types of stress incontinence are *urethral hypermobility* and *intrinsic sphincteric deficiency* (ISD).

In some instances when you have stress incontinence, poor support of the pelvic floor structures causes the urethra to move up and down rather than tightening when you cough or sneeze. This condition is called urethral hypermobility. In other cases, the urethral sphincter muscles have lost the ability to close tightly enough to prevent urine loss when you cough, sneeze, laugh, or exercise. This is referred to as intrinsic sphincteric deficiency (ISD). It is possible to have both urethral hypermobility and ISD at the same time. Surgical procedures used to treat stress incontinence include the injection of bulking agents, the use of radiofrequency energy, sling procedures, bladder neck suspension procedures, the insertion of an artificial sphincter, and pelvic organ prolapse repair procedures.

Injection of Bulking Agents

The injection of bulking agents is used in a minimally invasive procedure to treat stress incontinence. These materials are injected to bulk up or fill out the tissues surrounding the urethra in an effort to treat stress incontinence. Once materials are injected, they solidify into a spongy consistency that enhances urethral support and improves the urethra's ability to close tightly. Studies of bulking agents have shown a reduction in episodes of leakage when you cough, sneeze, laugh, or exercise.

Many materials are used as bulking agents, including those that follow.

Bovine Collagen

Collagen is a natural protein that is found in the skin, tendons, and bones of both humans and animals. FDA-approved bovine collagen is derived from purified collagen that comes from cows. Using bovine collagen as a bulking agent may produce an allergic reaction in some women. Therefore, you will need to have a skin test about four to six weeks prior to your procedure to determine if you are allergic to the material. For this test, a small amount of collagen is injected under the skin of your arm. If there are any signs of an allergic reaction during the four- to six-week test period, collagen implants may not be appropriate for you.

Carbon-Coated Beads

Carbon-coated beads are another injectable approved by the FDA for use as a bulking agent in the treatment of stress incontinence. The carbon-coated beads are suspended in a water-based gel. Carbon coating has been used in heart valve operations for decades and does not require a skin test. It is thought to provide longer-lasting results than bovine collagen agents.

Calcium Hydroxylapatite

A natural component of your teeth and bones, calcium hydroxylapatite is an FDA-approved bulking agent. Calcium hydroxylapatite is made of round particles suspended in a water-based gel. This agent does not require a skin test for allergies, and it may require fewer reinjections than other materials.

Autologous Fat

Fatty tissue taken from your own abdomen (autologous tissue) may be used as a bulking agent and does not require FDA approval. Using your own fat eliminates the risk of allergies that may occur when using other materials, such as bovine collagen. However, fat may be absorbed by the body at a rapid pace, which means results may not last as long as with other agents. This makes routine follow-up injections a necessity. Harvesting your own fat also requires a small incision in the lower abdomen and liposuction of a small amount of fat. Typically, only half an ounce to one ounce of fat is necessary for the procedure.

Undergoing a Bulking Agent Procedure

This minimally invasive procedure takes about fifteen minutes and may take place in a doctor's office or in an outpatient facility. Typically, a local anesthetic jelly is used to numb the urethra and bladder and may be combined with sedation to minimize discomfort. Local anesthetics are typically preferred because they leave you alert enough to provide feedback during the procedure. In some cases, regional or general anesthesia may be recommended.

Using a cystoscope to look inside the urethra, your physician will insert a needle either through the cystoscope or next to the urethra to inject the bulking agents in the urinary sphincter area. After the injections have been made, you may be asked to cough to determine whether the bulking agents are working. If you continue to leak, your physician may add further injections until you are able to cough without leaking. Being able to adjust the amount of bulking agents used during your procedure is key to achieving a good result.

Injection of Bulking Agents

Bulking agents, injected into the urethra, near the bladder neck, help close the urethra and prevent leakage. The bulking agents do not interfere with normal urination.

Recovery from a Bulking Agent Procedure

Usually, you will remain in the doctor's office or in a recovery room for no more than a few hours after your procedure. Before allowing you to leave, your physician will want to ensure that you are able to empty your bladder. In some cases, you may notice a little blood in the urine. This is common and is not a cause for concern. To prevent infection following your procedure, a three-day course of antibiotics is usually prescribed.

No bandages or dressings are required and, typically, you may resume your normal activities the following day. However, it is advised to avoid sexual intercourse for up to four weeks. Typically, results are noticeable immediately. In some instances, the effects of bulking agents may wear off after a couple of years. In this case, follow-up injections are necessary to maintain results.

Side Effects and Potential Complications

Side effects from a bulking agent procedure are typically minimal. Pain is usually mild and may be alleviated with over-the-counter pain remedies. You may also experience some pain or burning while urinating, but this is usually temporary and often goes away without treatment. Any blood that appears in your urine following the procedure should resolve in a few days.

Complications are uncommon but may include the following:

Urinary retention: An inability to empty your bladder may require you to perform self-catheterization until retention is resolved.

Urinary tract infection: If an infection occurs, you will likely be treated with antibiotics.

Urgency/frequency: A sense of urinary urgency may occur, and you may feel the need to urinate more frequently than usual.

Worsening of incontinence: It is possible, but unusual, that bulking agents will actually worsen incontinence symptoms.

Bulking agent migration: In rare cases, the bulking material may migrate to another area of the body, causing potentially serious complications.

Allergic reaction: If collagen is used, there is a risk for an allergic reaction.

Radiofrequency Energy

A minimally invasive procedure using radiofrequency energy (RF) may be recommended to treat stress incontinence. RF is used to heal tissues within the urinary tract. Once healed, the treated tissues are firmer and better able to withstand intraabdominal pressures caused by actions such as laughing, coughing, and sneezing.

Radiofrequency energy is available in an FDA-approved treatment called *Renessa.* A clinical trial has shown that more than three-fourths of women undergoing the Renessa procedure reported fewer episodes of incontinence, and more than one-third of women eliminated incontinence completely.

Undergoing Radiofrequency Energy Procedure

This procedure takes about thirty minutes and can be performed in your physician's office or in an outpatient facility. Local anesthesia may be combined with sedation for this procedure, which requires no incisions. The procedure involves passing a small probe through your urethra and into the bladder. A small balloon at the tip of the probe is inflated to keep the probe in the proper position.

Four small needles in the probe deliver RF to the tissues at the bladder neck and urethra for sixty seconds. After the sixty seconds, the probe is moved slightly and the needles deliver RF for an additional sixty seconds to another area of the bladder neck and urethra. RF is delivered a total of nine times during the procedure for sixty seconds each time. Once the tissues have been heated using a low temperature, the probe is removed and the procedure is over.

Recovery from a Radiofrequency Energy Procedure

In most cases, this minimally invasive procedure involves a speedy recovery. Because no incisions are made, no bandages or dressings are required. Limitations on your activities are minimal and, typically, you can return to your normal routine by the next day.

Side Effects and Potential Complications

Pain is usually minimal and may not require anything more than over-the-counter pain relievers. If your pain is not relieved with these drugs, stronger medications can be prescribed by your physician.

Sling Procedures

Sling procedures are the most common surgical option used to treat stress incontinence, and they may be performed on an outpatient basis or may require an overnight stay in the hospital. They may be used to treat both urethral hypermobility and intrinsic sphincteric deficiency (ISD), and their long-term success rate is about 85 percent. In sling operations, a narrow strip of material is placed within the pelvis to create a sling or hammock that supports the urethra and the bladder neck. The sling may be attached to the pubic bone, to ligaments, or to the connective tissues (fascia) of the lower abdomen and pelvis.

The additional support provided by slings helps keep the urethra closed when you exercise, cough, sneeze, or laugh. Studies show that these procedures are very effective in treating stress incontinence. In fact, sling operations offer a better long-term success rate than any other surgical procedure to treat stress incontinence.

Materials Used for Sling Procedures

A number of materials are used for slings, including synthetic materials, your own tissue (autologous tissue), tissue from a cadaver donor, and animal tissue.

Synthetic materials: A synthetic mesh is the most commonly used material in sling procedures. Available in a wide variety of shapes and sizes, synthetic mesh can be custom-fit for your individual anatomy. In some cases, synthetic mesh may erode or extrude, meaning the mesh may press through the adjacent tissues.

Autologous tissue: Using your own tissue requires an additional incision, usually in the lower abdomen or leg, to harvest the material. This may cause increased postoperative pain and recovery time. However, because the tissue is from your own body, there is no chance of it being rejected by your immune system.

Cadaveric tissue: When cadaveric tissue is used, you do not require any additional incisions. Tissue from cadaveric donors is typically well tolerated; however, in rare cases, it may break down. If this should occur, it can lead to recurrence of incontinence and additional surgery, with synthetic graft material, may be required.

Animal tissue: Typically, animal tissues are derived from pigs or cows. Porcine tissues generally work well as a sling material. Rarely, these tissues may break down, cause an immune reaction, reabsorb, or cause an infection. These materials do not require preoperative allergy testing.

Undergoing a Sling Procedure

Several variations of sling operations are used, but the basic procedure calls for the sling to be inserted through an incision in the vagina. This is called a *pubovaginal sling procedure.* The operation takes one to two hours and requires anesthesia. In many cases, this may be a combination of local anesthetic and IV sedation.

Depending on the type of sling procedure being performed, your operation may begin with the insertion of a

Sling Placement

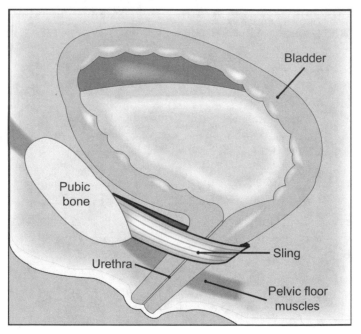

During a sling procedure, a physician secures a sling under the bladder and the urethra. The sling adds support and prevents leakage.

catheter into the urethra. In unusual cases, a suprapubic tube may be inserted into the bladder through a small incision in the lower abdomen. In many cases, no catheter is required.

Sling procedures may be performed using a variety of incisions and techniques. In some cases, the entire procedure may be completed through one or two vaginal incisions. In other cases, a combination of one vaginal incision and one incision in the lower abdomen may be used. In general, the sling is inserted through a vaginal incision and placed in a supportive position.

The sling may be secured to the pubic bone, to ligaments, or to the connective tissues of the lower abdomen and pelvis. When the sling is anchored to the pubic bone, tiny bone screws are passed through one of the incisions and secured to the underside of the pubic bone. Sutures may be used to attach the sling to ligaments or connective tissues.

Regardless of the placement of the incisions, your surgeon may use a cystoscope during the procedure to aid in the proper placement of the sling and screws or sutures. Once the sling has been secured, the incisions are closed and the operation is completed.

Recovery from a Sling Procedure

Following your operation, you will remain in the recovery room for a few hours. In some cases, you may require an overnight stay in the hospital. After a sling procedure, you will be instructed to limit your activity during the first few days and to rest often. Even though you will be limiting your activity, it is still important to get up and walk from time to time during this initial recovery period.

Typically, you will have to wait a couple of days after your operation before showering, and you will need to avoid swimming and taking baths for one to two weeks. Sexual activity is prohibited for approximately four to six weeks. To encourage proper healing, you should avoid rigorous exercise and heavy lifting for up to three months.

Using Catheters Following Sling Procedures

In most cases, if a catheter is used during your procedure, it will be removed before you return home. Usually, you will be asked to try to urinate in the recovery room or hospital, and once you are able to do so on your own, the catheter will be removed. On rare occasions, if you are not able to urinate normally, you may need to go home with the catheter in place. In this instance, before you go home you will receive specific instructions on how to empty your bladder using the catheter while your urinary tract continues to heal.

If you return home with a catheter, it will be left in place until your first follow-up appointment. It will be removed in your surgeon's office, and you will be instructed to try to urinate. If you are unable to, the catheter may be reinserted for an additional period of time. In some cases, if you are still unable to urinate on your own, you may be instructed how to catheterize yourself. You may also be asked to self-catheterize to measure the residual urine in your bladder after urinating.

Suprapubic tubes are rarely used during surgical procedures for incontinence, but if one is used during your procedure, it is typically removed before you go home. However, if you are unable to urinate on your own following your procedure, you may return home with the tube in place. In this case, you will receive specific instructions on how to use the tube for voiding. The device is removed in the physician's office during a postoperative visit, usually within five to seven days.

Side Effects and Potential Complications

Once you return home after your sling procedure, you may experience some pain at the incision sites, and you will likely experience some degree of swelling and bruising. Pain medication may be prescribed to alleviate any discomfort. It is also common to experience a sense of urinary urgency after the procedure, but this sensation is usually mild and typically resolves with time. In rare cases, urgency may be so severe that it leads to urge incontinence. When this occurs, medication can be prescribed to relax the bladder.

Complications from sling surgery are uncommon, but you should be aware of them.

Urinary retention: The inability to urinate on your own occurs in fewer than 5 percent of patients. In most cases, retention resolves with time. In rare instances when retention lingers, a corrective procedure may be necessary. For instance, if a sling is pulled too tight, it may lead to retention, and a secondary operation may be required to loosen it.

Urinary tract infection: It is possible to get an infection even though antibiotics are typically prescribed to prevent them. Urinary tract infections are the most common, and usually go away after you take antibiotics. In rare cases, an infection may cause fevers, chills, nausea, or dizziness. In this case, intravenous antibiotics may be required in a hospital setting.

Sling erosion: The sling may erode through surrounding tissues. In some cases, this may necessitate a corrective procedure.

Wound infection: Incision sites can become infected and may require antibiotics and wound care.

Blood loss: In about 1 to 2 percent of cases, blood loss may require a transfusion.

Deep venous thrombosis (DVT)/Pulmonary embolism: In very rare cases, a blood clot may develop in a leg vein (this is called deep venous thrombosis, or DVT), typically causing pain and swelling in the lower leg. Even more rare, a blood clot can travel through the veins and block part of the lungs (this is called a pulmonary embolism), causing symptoms of shortness of breath and perhaps chest pain. If you notice these symptoms, go immediately to an emergency room.

Hematoma: Blood that pools under the skin is called a hematoma. The blood is typically reabsorbed by the body over time.

Numbness/Lower extremity weakness: Procedures that require your legs to be elevated for long periods of time may result in temporary numbness or weakness in the legs.

Suprapubic tube injury: In rare instances, placement of a suprapubic tube may puncture one of your pelvic organs, requiring surgical correction.

Chronic pain: Any operation may result in chronic pain at the surgery site.

Variations of Sling Procedures

A minimally invasive midurethral sling (MIMUS) procedure is a variation of a basic sling operation that is gaining widespread acceptance and is being used more frequently. This operation uses a tension-free vaginal tape to create a supportive sling for the urethra. The narrow, ribbonlike strip of tape is slightly more than three inches in length and is made from a synthetic mesh that requires no screws or sutures for placement. Scar tissue forms around the mesh to secure it in place. Studies report that about 85 to 90 percent of patients undergoing the procedure experience improvement or a complete cure of stress incontinence.

The MIMUS procedure takes about thirty minutes in an outpatient setting. One of the advantages of MIMUS surgery is that it may be performed using only a local or regional anesthetic. In some cases, general anesthesia may be recommended. Using local or regional anesthesia has the advantage of allowing you to participate in during the procedure. With a MIMUS procedure, tiny incisions may be made in a variety of locations. One variation uses only vaginal incisions. Other variations involve one incision in the vagina and two incisions either in the lower abdomen or in the inner creases of the thighs.

Retropubic techniques involve the placement of the sling behind the pubic bone, the bony prominence you feel in the lowest part of your abdomen. With this method, the material must be positioned adjacent to where the pelvic organs lie. When inner thigh incisions are used, it is called the *transobturator technique.*

The tape is inserted through the vagina, positioned tension-free under the urethra, and pulled up through the other vaginal incisions or through the two abdominal or inner thigh incisions. At this point you may be asked to participate in the procedure. Your surgeon may ask you to cough to see whether or not the sling prevents leakage. This quick test allows the surgeon to make any necessary adjustments to the tape during your procedure. Once adequate support is achieved, the ends of the tape are snipped off just below the skin at the two incision sites. Then the incisions are closed, and the operation is over.

Recovery time is quicker with a MIMUS procedure than with traditional sling operations. In most cases, you will not require catheterization and will be able to urinate on your own immediately following the procedure. Usually, you may go home a few hours after the procedure and may be able to return to your normal activities the next day. However, it is advised to refrain from strenuous activities, heavy lifting, and sexual intercourse for four to six weeks.

MIMUS Procedure

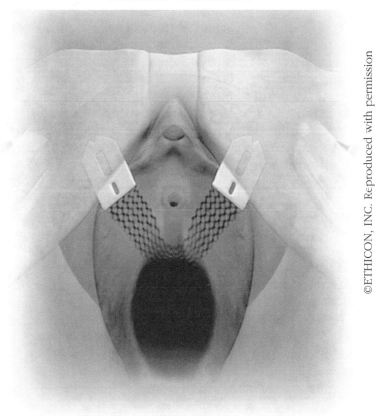

The minimally invasive midurethral sling (MIMUS) uses a mesh tape to support the urethra. The procedure helps prevent the accidental release of urine when a woman coughs, laughs, or moves vigorously or suddenly.

Bladder Neck Suspension Procedures

Bladder neck suspension is a surgical procedure that is typically used to treat stress incontinence caused by urethral hypermobility, a condition in which the urethra moves up and down rather than tightening when you cough or sneeze. The

American Urological Association Foundation has determined that bladder neck suspension procedures typically have poorer outcomes than sling procedures. Because of this, bladder neck suspension procedures are no longer commonly used, although some physicians still perform these operations.

The procedure may be performed on an outpatient or in-patient basis. Long-term success rates for these procedures are about 80 percent. As with sling procedures, bladder neck suspension provides support for the bladder neck and urethra. However, these procedures use different techniques to accomplish this goal.

Specifically, suspension operations use sutures rather than a sling to provide the necessary support. The sutures may be used to pull the bladder up from above, to lift it up from below, or a combination of these two methods. Typically, the sutures are placed between the ligaments and tendons that support the bladder and then tied to one of several possible supporting structures, including the pubic bone, fascia, or a ligament.

Bladder neck suspensions may be performed using vaginal incisions, abdominal incisions, or both. Procedures using vaginal incisions are referred to as needle suspension procedures, however this technique is rarely used anymore. Variations of the needle suspension technique include the Pereyra procedure, the Raz procedure, the Stamey procedure, and the Gittes procedure—named after the doctors who created them. When abdominal incisions are used, the procedure is called a retropubic suspension. Variations include the Burch and Marshall-Marchetti-Krantz procedures.

Undergoing a Bladder Neck Suspension

Bladder neck suspension procedures take about forty-five minutes to two hours depending on the technique used. General anesthesia and regional anesthesia are commonly used, but your surgeon may make a different recommendation. The procedure may begin with the insertion of a catheter. Next, vaginal incisions are made. In traditional retropubic procedures, the abdominal incision may measure about three to five inches long. Laparoscopic abdominal incisions measure about one-quarter of an inch.

Sutures are then passed through the incisions. Retropubic procedures call for the sutures to be inserted through the abdominal incision and secured to either ligaments or cartilage near the pubic bone. In needle suspension procedures, a long needle is used to pull the sutures from the vagina to the pubic bone or abdominal wall where they are anchored for support. Once the sutures have been secured, the incisions are closed.

Recovery from Bladder Neck Suspension

Following traditional bladder neck suspension procedure, you may require a night or two in the hospital. If you have a retropubic suspension procedure with wide abdominal incisions, you may be sent home with dressings on the wounds that must be changed on a daily basis. Your surgeon will provide information on how to care for your wounds while you heal.

In some cases, a catheter may remain in place for up to a few weeks after your procedure. The catheter is used to empty your bladder and will be removed in your doctor's office. Showering is allowed approximately two days after your procedure. Typically, you may return to your normal activities and to work within one to two weeks. However, it is recommended that you avoid heavy lifting and strenuous activities for up to four to six weeks. In fact, you may be instructed to permanently avoid lifting anything over twenty-five pounds because it may stretch or weaken the surgical repairs. In general, you must wait about one month before resuming sexual intercourse.

Side Effects and Potential Complications

After bladder neck suspension surgery, side effects may occur. For instance, it is common to feel some soreness in the pelvic area. Painkillers may be prescribed to minimize your discomfort. Following removal of the catheter, you may experience a sense of urgency or a burning sensation when you urinate. This typically goes away after a week or two.

Complications are rare but may include the following:

Urinary retention: When you are unable to urinate on your own, it is called urinary retention. This is typically a result of overcorrection during the procedure and may require adjustment in a secondary operation.

Injury to surrounding nerves or organs: As the sutures are passed through the pelvic area, damage to nerves or organs may occur. This may result in intrinsic sphincteric deficiency (ISD).

Poor wound healing: In some cases, you may require additional wound care if your wounds do not heal properly.

Vaginal prolapse: It is possible to experience vaginal prolapse following a bladder neck procedure. Correcting this problem may require another surgery.

Artificial Sphincter

Another procedure, artificial sphincter surgery, is an operation in which an inflatable artificial sphincter is inserted around the urethra to treat stress incontinence. This procedure is more common in men and rarely used in women, but may be a last-resort option for some women. An artificial sphincter is comprised of three parts: an inflatable cuff that is placed around the urethra, a pump that inflates the cuff, and a small balloon that regulates pressure. When you need to urinate, you press the pump and fluid placed in the cuff flows to the balloon, allowing the urethra to open so urine can drain out. The fluid automatically returns to the cuff after about ninety seconds, causing the urethra to close tightly.

This procedure is typically reserved for severe cases of stress incontinence and may be recommended if you have intrinsic sphincteric deficiency (ISD). Artificial sphincters have proven to be highly effective, with studies reporting a 92 percent cure rate in women with the device.

Undergoing an Artificial Sphincter Procedure

This procedure takes one to two hours and typically requires general or regional anesthesia. To begin your procedure, the surgeon inserts a catheter. An abdominal incision is made, and the balloon is passed through it and filled with fluid. The cuff is inserted through the same incision and positioned around the bladder neck. A tube is routed from the cuff to the balloon, and the pump is placed in the labia. Typically, your surgeon will remove the catheter and test the device before re-inserting the catheter and closing the incisions to finish the operation.

Recovery from an Artificial Sphincter Procedure

Recovering from an artificial sphincter operation takes time. Typically, you will be required to remain in the hospital for a few days following your procedure. The catheter is usually removed before you return home. Antibiotics are typically prescribed postoperatively to prevent infection.

In general, your body needs about six to eight weeks of healing time before the cuff is activated. You will be instructed to refrain from vigorous activity, heavy lifting, and sexual intercourse during this time. Your surgeon may recommend using protection products to cope with your incontinence symptoms during this period. Once your body has healed sufficiently, you will receive training on how to use the artificial sphincter. Proper usage of the device is key to its effectiveness.

Side Effects and Potential Complications

It is common to feel some pain and tenderness at the surgical site following your procedure. Pain medication may be prescribed to alleviate any discomfort. Complications are uncommon but may include the following:

Urinary retention: When this occurs, it may be caused by a kink in the tube or by an obstruction. Repair may require a minor surgical revision to correct the tubing problem.

Mechanical failure: In rare cases, the cuff may leak or malfunction. An obstruction may also occur within the system. These rare conditions all require surgical revision.

Migration of the cuff or pump: It is possible for the cuff or pump to migrate from its proper position within the body. A secondary procedure is necessary to correct migration.

Tissue atrophy: With time, the tissues underneath the cuff may begin to waste away. This prevents the cuff from closing the urethra tightly enough and may bring about a recurrence of incontinence. Tissue atrophy is the most common cause for surgical revision.

Urethral erosion: The cuff may erode the tissues of the urethra. In some cases, you may be instructed to deactivate the cuff at nighttime to reduce the risk of erosion.

Cuff erosion: Reported in 1 to 3 percent of patients, cuff erosion requires the removal of the cuff in a secondary procedure. A new cuff may be inserted approximately three to six months later in a surgical procedure.

Pelvic Organ Prolapse Repair

Surgical procedures that repair pelvic organ prolapse may also treat stress incontinence. Pelvic organ prolapse repair procedures are used to correct bladder prolapse *(cystocele)*, rectal prolapse *(rectocele)*, small bowel prolapse *(enterocele)*, and vaginal vault prolapse. The operation returns the organ to a more normal position within the pelvic area and strengthens surrounding structures.

Undergoing Pelvic Organ Prolapse Repair

Pelvic organ prolapse repair procedures take anywhere from thirty minutes to more than an hour and typically require general or regional anesthesia. Your operation will begin with the placement of a catheter. Incisions are made within the vagina and may also be made in the crease where your thigh meets your buttock or in the middle of your buttock.

For bladder prolapse, a supportive material, such as a synthetic mesh or biologic tissue graft, is positioned between the bladder and the vaginal wall to provide support. For procedures done to correct rectal prolapse, the material is placed between the rectum and the vaginal wall. When repairing vaginal vault prolapse, the material is secured at the upper end of the vagina to hold it in place. Once the material is secured in place, with permanent sutures, the incisions are closed and the operation is completed.

Laparoscopic Pelvic Organ Prolapse Procedures

In some cases, pelvic organ prolapse may be repaired laparoscopically. Typically, laparoscopic repairs take somewhat longer to perform than other procedures. In this surgery, small keyhole incisions are made in the abdomen and a slender tube with a camera at the tip is placed in one of the incisions to allow the surgeon to see the abdominal cavity. The prolapsed organ or organs are suspended using sutures and either synthetic mesh or a biological tissue graft. The incisions are closed and the operation is completed.

Recovery from Pelvic Organ Prolapse Repair

Following your pelvic organ repair operation, you may require an overnight stay in the hospital. During this time, you may be given nutrients, fluids, and medications through an IV in your arm. Typically, you may begin resuming your normal diet within a day or two. To avoid constipation after your procedure, you may be advised to take suppositories or a stool softener for several days.

Often, the catheter will be removed before you return home and you will be able to urinate on your own. In some cases, the catheter will remain in place for a few days. Incisions are usually small and heal quickly. Returning to work may take one to two weeks, depending on the nature of your work. It is advised to avoid vigorous exercise, heavy lifting, and sexual intercourse for up to eight weeks.

Side Effects and Potential Complications

Side effects associated with pelvic organ repairs include pain at the surgical site. Pain medication may be prescribed to diminish soreness. You may notice blood-tinged urine, but this normally resolves within a few days. Complications are uncommon but include:

Bleeding: As with any surgical procedure, excessive bleeding may occur.

Infection: In case of an infection, antibiotics will be administered.

Adjacent tissue/organ injury: In rare instances, tissues or organs near the prolapsed organ may be injured during the procedure. This may be corrected immediately during your operation or in a follow-up procedure.

Incontinence: In some cases, correcting pelvic organ prolapse can reveal other urinary problems, such as urethral hypermobility, which can cause stress incontinence. Often, this condition can be detected and corrected during your prolapse repair procedure.

Urinary retention: As with any pelvic surgery, swelling may cause temporary urinary retention.

Surgery for Urge Incontinence and Overactive Bladder

A growing number of procedures are being used to treat urge incontinence and overactive bladder. In many cases, they may advised if conservative therapies and medications have failed. In other instances, you may opt for surgical treatment instead of other treatment options. Procedures that may treat these conditions include sacral nerve stimulation and Botox injections. Other procedures, such as bladder augmentation, urinary diversion, and bladder denervation, are used infrequently, but may be an option for you.

Sacral Nerve Stimulation (InterStim Therapy)

InterStim Therapy involves implanting a small device that sends mild electrical pulses to a sacral nerve. As explained earlier, the sacral nerve sends signals to the bladder muscle when it is time to urinate. If you have urinary retention, overactive bladder, or urge incontinence, the sacral nerve may be sending signals at inappropriate times or may not be sending signals when necessary. InterStim Therapy changes the way the signal is transmitted between the sacral nerve and the spinal cord to improve urinary storage or emptying.

InterStim Therapy

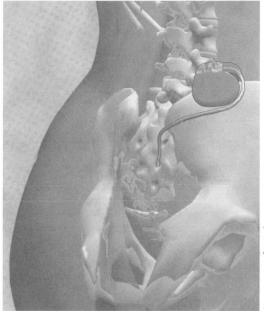

Courtesy of Medtronic, Inc.

The InterStim Therapy uses a transmitter that sends mild electrical pulses to the sacral nerve, in the lower back. This nerve effects the bladder and surrounding muscles that manage urinary function. The device is implanted under the skin in the upper buttocks or abdomen.

InterStim Therapy has proven effective in several clinical studies, which indicate that 45 percent of patients with urge incontinence remained completely dry following implantation, and 34 percent experienced at least a 50 percent reduction in leaking. For patients with urgency, 82 percent experienced a reduction in symptoms. Sixty-four percent of patients with frequency reduced the number of times they urinated. And 61 percent of patients with urinary retention eliminated the need for a catheter.

Undergoing a Sacral Nerve Stimulation Procedure

The surgical procedure for InterStim Therapy is a two-step process. First, a temporary test is performed to provide a preview of the kind of results you might expect from the procedure. This outpatient procedure takes one to two hours and is usually performed using a local anesthetic. Sedation may also be used in some instances.

This procedure requires two to three small incisions measuring just one to one and a half inches. The first incision is placed near the sacral nerve just above the tailbone. A thin wire lead with electrodes at the tip is passed through the incision using a needle and is placed near the sacral nerve. At this point during the procedure, you may be asked if you are feeling any sensations in the vaginal area. Your responses will help guide your surgeon in the proper placement of the lead during the implantation process. The lead is connected to an external device that provides mild stimulation. This device is carried in a small portable pouch.

During a period of three days to two weeks after the procedure, you will be asked to keep a bladder diary, noting any symptoms of urgency, frequency, or retention. After the test period, you and your physician will review your bladder diary. If the test shows improvement in your condition, your physician may recommend permanent implantation of the device. If improvement is minimal, the device may not be right for you.

Permanent implantation of the InterStim device takes less than an hour and is usually performed on an outpatient basis using a local anesthetic. In this simple procedure, a small incision is made in the upper buttock and a "pocket" is created. The doctor places a small neurostimulator device about the size of a stopwatch into the pocket under the skin. Then, working under the skin, the doctor connects the same lead that was used to test the device. All incisions are stitched up, bandages are applied, and the operation is completed. With this procedure, all parts of the device and lead are contained within the body. There are no wires or elements that can be seen externally.

Recovery from a Sacral Nerve Procedure

After the operation, you can expect to spend up to a few hours in the recovery room before going home. At home, you should take it easy for the first three to six weeks while your body heals. Following implantation, you will likely need to visit your surgeon a few times to fine-tune the stimulation settings. Using a handheld device to control the stimulation, your surgeon will test a range of safe settings. On your own, you can easily adjust the settings within that range using your own handheld device. Once you have your settings, you will probably only need to visit your doctor for checkups once or twice a year.

Side Effects and Potential Complications

Pain at the implant site is common following the procedure, and painkillers may be prescribed. Aside from pain felt after implantation, possible side effects include migration of the lead and infection.

Living with a Sacral Nerve Stimulator

Having a neurotransmitter implanted in your body may require you to make a few adjustments in your daily lifestyle. For instance, you may need to turn off the stimulator when you operate a vehicle, or if you use power tools.

When seeing a doctor or dentist, always inform the staff of your neurotransmitter because some medical equipment may interfere with the electrical pulses. Likewise, if you are ever admitted to the hospital or emergency room, it is very important to provide information about your device. For this purpose, you will receive an identification card that includes information about your sacral nerve stimulator along with your doctor's contact information. If you prefer, you may choose to wear a medical alert bracelet with this information.

The neurotransmitter typically lasts about seven to ten years before the battery runs down. At that time, if you want to continue the therapy, you can choose to replace it with a new device in an outpatient procedure. During this procedure, your surgeon will also check that the lead and other components are working properly. If they aren't, they will be replaced with new parts.

Special Considerations about InterStim Therapy

You should be aware that InterStim Therapy implantation is expensive and can cost as much as $20,000 when you include doctor's fees, operating room costs, and the price of the device. InterStim Therapy is usually covered by insurance.

Botulinum Toxin Type A (Botox) Injections

Botox injections are a minimally invasive procedure used to treat overactive bladder and urge incontinence. Botox is a neurotoxin that blocks nerve transmissions to muscles. It earned FDA approval in 2002 as a drug that can reduce the appearance of facial frown lines. Injecting Botox into the bladder to provide relief for symptoms of overactive bladder or urge incontinence is considered an off-label usage of the drug.

Botox injections into the bladder have shown a decrease in bladder contractions and a reduction in leakage. In fact, one study showed a significant increase in the amount of urine the bladder could hold and an average decrease in daytime bathroom trips from twelve to four.

Undergoing a Botox Injection Procedure

Botox injections are typically an office-based procedure that takes less than thirty minutes. To minimize discomfort, a local anesthetic in the form of a numbing gel is applied to the urethra. A local anesthetic may also be injected into the bladder. A cystoscope—a long, thin instrument with a tiny camera on the tip—is inserted through the urethra into the bladder. A needle is then inserted through the cystoscope, and the Botox injections are made in the bladder. After approximately twenty to thirty injections have been made, the needle and cystoscope are removed to complete the procedure.

Recovering from Your Botox Injections Procedure

You may need to remain in your physician's office for about fifteen minutes after your injections. Following the procedure, there are no restrictions on your activities. You may drive home or return to work if necessary. To prevent infection following the procedure, you may be instructed to take an antibiotic for a few days.

Side Effects and Potential Complications

Few side effects or complications are associated with Botox injections in the bladder. Some mild soreness may be felt, but can usually be managed with over-the-counter pain relievers. In extremely rare cases, temporary urinary retention may result. If this occurs, you will be instructed how to perform intermittent catheterization to drain urine from the bladder.

Special Considerations about Botox Injections

While Botox injections may be effective, they are also expensive. The injections typically cost approximately $500–$1,000 per session, and they are not covered by insurance. In addition, the results may last only six to nine months. This means you need to continue getting the injections on an ongoing basis in order to maintain positive results.

Bladder Augmentation

Bladder augmentation is a major surgical procedure that increases the size of the bladder. This procedure is performed very infrequently to treat incontinence, but may be considered an option for you. Typically, bladder augmentation is accomplished by adding a segment of the bowel, small intestine, or stomach, to the bladder.

Preparing for Bladder Augmentation

If a portion of your bowel will be used to augment your bladder, you will need to prepare for the procedure. Bowel prep is typically required to cleanse the area thoroughly in an effort to prevent infection during the operation. In most cases,

121

you will be instructed to follow a low-fiber diet for a few days preoperatively and to eat nothing except clear liquids the day before your procedure.

The day before your operation, you may be asked to complete a bowel preparation at home. Or, once at the hospital, you may be asked to drink a strong laxative that is used to clean out the bowel. In some cases, this laxative may be administered through a tube in your nose. This laxative will cause you to have several loose stools. After approximately four to six hours, the stools should be clear and watery, signaling that your bowel is ready for the augmentation procedure. Most individuals complete preoperative bowel preparations as outpatients.

Undergoing Bladder Augmentation

A bladder augmentation procedure takes about three hours and typically requires general anesthesia. To begin the operation, a catheter and a suprapubic tube are inserted. Then a vertical incision is made from the belly button down to the pubic hair. The top of the bladder is opened with an incision. A section of the bowel, small intestine, or stomach is removed and used as a patch on the top of the bladder and affixed in place using sutures or staples. The area where the tissue was removed is also closed with sutures or staples. The abdominal incision is closed to complete the operation.

Recovery from Bladder Augmentation

Bladder augmentation is considered major surgery, and recovery will take time. Following your operation, you may be required to remain in the hospital for up to two weeks. You will not be allowed to eat or drink anything for as much as one week after your procedure. All fluids, nutrients, and medications will be given via an IV tube in your arm. Your specialist will determine when you are able to begin drinking and eating solid food again. You will most likely be told to follow a special diet for a few months. It may be several months before you can return to work.

A catheter or suprapubic tube may remain in place for several weeks following your procedure. Tests to ensure that the augmented bladder is leak-proof will be performed before the drainage device is removed. While your bladder is healing, you may be instructed to take medication that relaxes the bladder, along with antibiotics to prevent infection.

Side Effects and Potential Complications

Pain is a common complaint following bladder augmentation, but typically can be controlled with prescription medication. Passing blood in the urine or experiencing painful urination is common but usually temporary.

Complications are rare, but include the following:

Perforation of the bladder: Medical experts aren't sure what causes a perforation of the bladder, but it may cause symptoms of nausea, pain, and bloating. The condition requires surgical correction.

Deep venous thrombosis (DVT): A blood clot that may occur deep in the leg as a result of surgery.

Infection: Even though antibiotics are used, an infection may occur.

Incontinence: In some cases, you may experience temporary incontinence while your body heals.

Nocturia: Nighttime incontinence may occur as a result of the procedure.

Blockage or rupture of organs: In extremely rare instances, a blockage may develop in the intestine or kidney, or the bladder may rupture. Symptoms of such a condition include sudden pain, vomiting, nausea, and fever. These conditions are considered medical emergencies. If you experience these symptoms, go immediately to an emergency room.

Bladder stones: It is possible for stones to develop in the bladder.

Bladder cancer: In extremely rare cases, bladder cancer may develop after bladder augmentation. Statistics show a 1.2 percent risk. Accordingly, any woman who undergoes this procedure should be checked regularly so that the development of any cancer can be detected early. This means having annual bladder exams (cystoscopy) and urine sample testing after the augmentation surgery and having biopsies performed ten years after the surgery.

Diarrhea: Chronic diarrhea may occur when segments of the bowel are used to augment the bladder.

Urinary Diversion Surgery

In extremely rare cases, when all attempts to alleviate your incontinence symptoms have failed, a major surgical procedure called urinary diversion may be used. In this uncommon procedure, the flow of urine is rerouted away from the normal urinary tract structures.

In some cases, a replacement bladder is fashioned out of the intestine. In other cases, urine is diverted from the urinary tract to a hole that is created in the abdominal wall. The urine either drains from the hole into an ostomy bag that must be worn at all times, or is drained using a tube. An ostomy bag is a pouch that is worn outside the body to collect urine as it drains from the body.

Preparing for a Urinary Diversion Procedure

In some cases, you will need to undergo certain preoperative preparations. For instance, if any portion of your bowel is to be used in your operation, bowel prep will be required. Typically, you will go to the hospital the day before your procedure where you will take a strong laxative to cleanse your bowel in an effort to prevent infection. As mentioned previously, most bowel preparations are done on an outpatient basis.

Undergoing Urinary Diversion

Urinary diversion operations are performed using general anesthesia and take about two to four hours. An incision is made in the abdomen to begin the procedure. The ureters are cut free from the bladder. Depending on the underlying problem, the bladder may be removed or left in the body. In some procedures, the ureters will be attached to a portion of the intestine, which is then brought through the abdominal wall. In other cases, a replacement bladder is created using portions of the small or large intestine. The ureters are attached to the new bladder. In some cases, a small incision designed to be a permanent opening will be made in the lower abdomen. This permanent opening is called a stoma.

Recovery from Urinary Diversion

Because urinary diversion is considered major surgery, it requires a lengthy recovery. A hospital stay of up to ten days is to be expected. During your initial hospital stay, you will receive all fluids and nutrients through an IV in your arm. When your surgeon determines that you are ready to resume your diet, you will begin with liquids only and progress to solid foods.

When you return home, you may have urinary stomal diversion stents or a stomal catheter in place for several weeks. Stents are tubes that go from the stoma up into the ureters. Your surgeon will determine when these tubes can be removed. Removal is performed during an office visit.

Side Effects and Potential Complications

You should expect to feel some pain at the abdominal incision site. Prescription drugs can help alleviate this pain during your recovery.

Complications may include the following:

Bleeding: As with any major surgery, excessive bleeding is a possibility.

Infection: Although rare, infection may occur. Typically, it can be treated with antibiotics.

Deep venous thrombosis (DVT)/Pulmonary embolism: A blood clot may develop deep in the leg (this is called deep venous thrombosis, or DVT), causing pain, swelling, and redness, often in the calf. In rare cases, a blood clot may travel to the lungs (this is called a pulmonary embolism), causing shortness of breath. Proceed immediately to an emergency room if you experience these symptoms.

Stomal complications: Tissue death due to inadequate blood supply may require a revisionary procedure. Narrowing of the opening due to scarring or infection may be corrected in a minor procedure. A small hernia caused by the bowel bulging into the abdominal wall may be managed with additional ostomy supplies; however, a larger hernia may require a surgical repair.

Metabolic imbalance: Urinary diversion procedures may cause an imbalance in your fluid or salt levels.

Bowel problems: Bowel obstruction or bowel leakage may occur. In such cases, your physician has several treatment options. You may need to fast, be fed intravenously, or have a nasogastric decompression tube inserted; this flexible suction tube is inserted through a nostril into the intestinal track, where it decompresses gas and liquid, helping to prevent leakage. Other cases may require a return to surgery to correct the problem.

Coping After a Urinary Diversion

If you require an ostomy bag as a result of your urinary diversion procedure, you and your family members will receive detailed instructions on how you will use it. In some cases, once you return home, a therapist who specializes in such matters will assist you in learning how to use the bag. Over time, you will become accustomed to using the bag and, in most cases, should be able to resume all your daily activities.

Bladder Denervation

Used only in extremely rare situations, denervation is a surgical procedure that severs the sacral nerves that supply the bladder. This procedure is usually reserved for incontinence cases that are accompanied by severe, chronic pain. Denervation may alleviate the pain, but it destroys bladder function, leaving you totally incontinent. Lifelong self-catheterization or use of diapers is required following the procedure.

Chapter 7

Living with Incontinence

Even if you see improvement in your symptoms thanks to conservative therapy, medication, or surgery, you may still need a little help staying dry from time to time. Or, if you are still waiting for treatment to produce positive results, you may want some protection in the meantime. Fortunately, there are hundreds of personal products and medical devices that can help.

Thanks to these easy-to-use items, you may be encouraged to resume some of your favorite activities, such as social events and physical exercise. Available either over-the-counter or with a prescription, these products can help you resume a normal lifestyle.

Medical Devices

Medical devices that treat incontinence include urethral devices, pessaries, and catheters. Some of these devices are inserted into the vagina or urethra. Others are used on the exterior of the urethra. In general, medical devices are worn to prevent leakage or to provide support for the pelvic organs. Some are designed to treat stress incontinence; others may alleviate symptoms associated with stress or urge incontinence.

In some cases, you may experience immediate relief from symptoms when wearing one of these devices. They may be used whether you are looking for a long-term solution or just temporary help while you wait for more long-lasting results from other treatment options. Your physician can determine if you might benefit from wearing a medical device and can give you a prescription.

Urethral Inserts

Urethral inserts are narrow tubes that are placed inside the urethra to prevent urinary leakage. Designed to treat stress incontinence, these devices are known as *occlusive devices* because they block urine from escaping. Inserts may also be called urethral plugs and are available with a prescription from your physician. Two urethral inserts are available: Reliance Urinary Control Insert Device and FemSoft. The Reliance device earned FDA approval in 1996 and is widely available, whereas the FemSoft insert is newer on the market.

The Reliance device is inserted into the urethra using a reusable syringe. At the tip of the tube is a small balloon that inflates after insertion to block urine from escaping. On the other end of the tube is a string that is used to pull the device out each time you need to urinate. When you pull the string, the balloon deflates, facilitating removal of the device. The used device is thrown away and replaced with a new one.

FemSoft is a silicone tube that is wrapped with a soft silicone sleeve filled with mineral oil. The device is inserted into the urethra using a disposable applicator. Once it is in place, the sleeve expands to form a balloon that seals the urethra to prevent leakage. On the other end of the tube is small tab that is used for easy removal when you need to urinate. After urination, you simply dispose of the tube and insert a new one.

These devices come in a variety of sizes to fit women of every shape and size. For this reason, you must visit your physician for a fitting before using a urethral insert. In many cases, your doctor will show you how to insert and remove the device. Even with this instruction, it may take some time for you to feel comfortable using the insert.

It is recommended that you replace the inserts at least every six hours and remove them at night. In addition, the inserts should be removed during sexual intercourse. Using urethral inserts may cause side effects, including bacteria in the urine, urinary tract infection, frequency, and urgency.

Urethral Pads

Urethral pads are single-use foam patches that are placed on the exterior of the urethra to prevent stress incontinence. Known as occlusive devices, these pads are designed to block urine from leaking rather than to absorb urine that has already leaked from the bladder. Slightly larger and thicker than a quarter and somewhat triangular in shape, each patch has an adhesive substance on one side that sticks to the urethra, creating a seal. When you are ready to urinate, you remove the patch and dispose of it. After urinating, you replace the old patch with a new one.

During vigorous exercise, the patch may shift slightly. Pads can be worn for up to five hours during the day and can be worn throughout the night. However, urethral pads should not be worn during sexual intercourse. Likewise, avoid using the patch if you have a urinary or vaginal infection. Sold under the brand name Impress Softpatch, the FDA-approved urethral pads are available without a prescription in most drugstores.

Urethral Shields

Urethral shields are FDA-approved devices that use suction to prevent stress, urge, or mixed incontinence. The suction helps tighten the urethra and keeps it closed to avoid leakage. Made of silicone, these small, round shields are about the size of a quarter. An adhesive gel is applied to the side that is placed over the urethra to create a seal. When you need to urinate, you remove the shield and wash it with soap and water before reapplying it. You may continue using the same shield for up to seven days.

FemAssist and CapSure, two brands of urethral shields, are available with a prescription. Studies of urethral shields have shown that they are both safe and effective. Side effects have been noted with the reusable shields, including skin irritations and urinary tract infections.

Pessaries

A pessary is a small, silicone or latex device that is placed inside the vagina to prevent stress incontinence. Pessaries are FDA-approved and may also be used to provide support for pelvic organs, such as the bladder, uterus, or rectum. For the treatment of stress incontinence, a pessary presses against the urethra and elevates the bladder neck. This allows the urethra to close more completely to prevent involuntary loss of urine.

These devices come in a wide variety of sizes and shapes, but pessaries that treat stress incontinence are usually shaped like a ring or a dish. For better support, a cube-shaped pessary may be recommended if you experience incontinence only during vigorous exercise, such as jogging or aerobics. Another pessary that may be recommended to treat stress incontinence is called Introl and it has a round shape with two prongs that provide support for the bladder neck. If you have pelvic organ prolapse in addition to incontinence, a different style of pessary, one shaped like a bar-bell, may offer the most support.

Pessaries are available with a prescription and must be fitted in a physician's office. Fitting is typically accomplished by trial and error, and you may need to experiment with a few different sizes before finding the pessary that works best for you. In most cases, you will be asked to return to your doctor's office for regular follow-up visits to determine how well your pessary is working for you.

In some cases, your doctor will provide instructions on how to insert, remove, and clean the pessary yourself. For example, if you have exercise-induced incontinence, you may be instructed to insert the pessary prior to exercise and to remove it and clean it with soap and water once you have finished your workout. For other types of stress incontinence, you may leave the pessary in place for days or weeks at a time before removing it and cleaning it. Some pessaries require routine care in a medical office every few months rather than self-care.

When a pessary is inserted properly, it should not cause any discomfort or any difficulty urinating. You should alert your physician if your pessary causes any pain or prevents you from urinating normally. In general, pessaries are not advised if you have a vaginal infection. In some cases, pessaries may cause vaginal irritation, discharge, or odor. A vaginal estrogen cream may be recommended to minimize these side effects.

Summary of Treatment Options

Stress Incontinence	Overactive Bladder/ Urge Incontinence	Overflow/ Incontinence
Pelvic floor therapy	Pelvic floor therapy	Medication
Bladder training	Bladder training	Sacral nerve stimulator implants
Lifestyle changes	Timed voiding	Self-catheterization
Urethral inserts	Lifestyle changes	Surgery
Urethral pads	Urethral shields	
Urethral shields	Biofeedback	
Pessaries	Electrical stimulation	
Biofeedback	Medication	
Electrical stimulation	Botox injections	
Medication	Sacral nerve stimulator implants	
Bulking agents	Surgery	
Radiofrequency energy		
Surgery		

Catheters

A catheter is a narrow, hollow tube that is inserted into the urethra and up into the bladder to empty the bladder. Using a catheter can reduce urinary leakage by keeping your bladder empty. In some cases, your doctor may recommend temporary self-catheterization, which may also be called intermittent self-catheterization. A wide variety of catheters are available for this use with a prescription. Your physician will provide instructions on how and when to perform self-catheterization.

Typically, you will be required to insert a catheter every three to six hours to empty your bladder. It is important to wash your hands with warm soapy water before and after you perform self-catheterization.

You should also clean the urethra using a moist towelette prior to inserting the catheter. Applying a water-soluble lubricant to the catheter may facilitate insertion. Once you are prepared, insert the catheter slowly into the urethra until urine begins to flow through the tube. Keep it in place until the urine stops and then slowly remove the catheter.

It's also important to keep the catheter clean. Between uses, you can soak it in Betadine, a sterile iodine solution, or you can sterilize it by putting it water and bringing it to a boil on the stove top or in a microwave oven. Make sure the device has cooled completely before using.

For convenience in using the catheter away from home, you can carry your catheters with you in a zip-style plastic bag, a toothbrush holder, or a tote designed specifically for the devices. Few risks are associated with temporary catheterization, but you should notify your doctor if you notice cloudy or foul-smelling urine, if you feel pain when trying to insert the catheter, or if the catheter won't insert easily.

Neuromodulation Devices

These devices, which provide nerve stimulation, may be used to treat urge incontinence and overactive bladder. The sacral nerve, which is located in the sacrum at the lower end of the spine, signals the bladder when it is time to urinate. Sometimes, this nerve sends out signals too frequently, causing symptoms of urge incontinence or overactive bladder. Neuromodulation devices can reduce the number of signals being sent to the bladder, thereby reducing these symptoms.

The Urgent PC Neuromodulation System affects the sacral nerve through percutaneous tibial nerve stimulation (PTNS). The tibial nerve is located just above the ankles but is connected to the sacral nerve. In this minimally invasive office-based procedure, a needle is inserted just above the ankle. An electrode connected to the needle sends an electrical current through the nervous system. Other than the slight prick of the needle, PTNS should be painless.

Studies have shown a success rate of 60 to 80 percent using PTNS, with significant reductions in frequency and episodes of leakage. To benefit from PTNS, you will need to have a series of about twelve weekly sessions lasting thirty minutes each. After the initial program, you will require follow-up sessions from time to time.

■ When are medical devices recommended?

Medical devices may be advised in numerous situations. For instance, if you continue to have troublesome incontinence despite trying pelvic floor therapy, these devices may provide some necessary relief. In addition, if you only leak during certain activities, such as high-intensity exercise, a device may help keep you dry.

Medical devices may offer temporary relief of your symptoms while you wait for a convenient time to schedule surgery for a permanent repair. Similarly, if you are a candidate for surgery but are planning on having children in the future, you may benefit from a medical device. As explained previously, childbirth can reverse the repairs achieved in surgery, making it is advisable to postpone surgical procedures until after you have finished having children. In the meantime, a medical device may alleviate your symptoms. In addition, if you would simply prefer to avoid surgery, or if you are deemed unfit for surgery, medical devices offer an alternative treatment option.

Personal Products

Hundreds of personal care products are available to help you cope with episodes of incontinence. Most products are designed to help keep your skin and clothing dry while reducing odors associated with involuntary urine loss. The products that will work best for you depend on the level of absorbency you need. Your doctor may be able to assist you in choosing personal care products that will meet your needs. In general, these products fall into a few product categories, including pads, undergarments, skin protectants, and odor control.

Pads

Disposable absorbent pads are the most common personal care product used for incontinence. Disposable pads are no bulkier than those used for menstruation, but are far more absorbent and better at keeping you and your clothing dry. Available in dozens of shapes and sizes, pads can be worn under everyday clothing and can be used whether leakage is light, moderate, or severe. Pads are typically made of three layers. The top layer wicks moisture away from your body. The middle layer locks in liquid. The bottom layer is usually waterproof, preventing urine from leaking onto your clothing. Many pads also offer odor control.

Undergarments

If you have a high level of leakage, you may want to use disposable or reusable diapers or special underwear that is designed to handle urine loss. Disposable diapers are typically available in sizes small, medium, large, and extra large. In general, you should look for a snug fit when choosing a size. Disposable diapers are popular due to their convenience, but that convenience can be expensive.

Reusable diapers tend to look more like underwear and have a waterproof crotch where a reusable pad or panty liner is attached. Some reusable undergarments resemble normal underwear but offer the same absorbency as a diaper. Designed with a special material in the crotch that wicks moisture away from the body, these undergarments provide discreet protection in a variety of absorbency levels. With these undergarments, you do not need to wear an additional pad or panty liner.

Other reusable products include belted undergarments and washable cloth diapers. Belted undergarments are designed for moderate to heavy leakage. Disposable shields are used with the reusable belts. Cloth diapers are typically worn under a plastic cover to prevent urine from soiling your clothing.

Skin Protectants

A number of products can be used to help prevent skin irritations, which may occur when urine comes into prolonged contact with the skin. Products such as wet wipes, cleansers, barrier creams, moisturizers, ointments, and powders may help protect your skin by keeping it clean and dry. Look for products that are designed specifically to protect skin from irritations caused by incontinence and use them as directed. Overuse of some products may also irritate your skin.

Odor Control

Several products, including sprays and tablets, are available to help you remain odor-free when leakage occurs. Sprays may be applied directly to absorbent pads or diapers to remove odors. Deodorant tablets are taken orally like a vitamin and reduce embarrassing odors.

■ How do I decide which type of product is best for me?

In general, the level of protection you require will dictate which products will best fit your needs. For instance, if you only dribble when you sneeze or cough, you may need nothing more than an incontinence panty liner for protection. If you leak heavy doses of urine, however, you will need more-substantial protection, such as an adult diaper or undergarment. The right personal care products for you also depend on your personal preference. You may need to try a few brands or styles before finding the products that are both comfortable and provide adequate protection.

■ Where can I purchase incontinence care supplies?

Many of these products can be purchased in your local drugstore, from online retailers, or through specialty catalogs. Online sellers and specialty catalogs tend to offer a wider variety of products, including hard-to-find brands, than what you might find in your local store. Some online stores also offer samples of their absorbent products so you can test them before purchasing a large quantity.

■ What are some tips for making it through everyday trips and errands?

A little preparation can help you remain dry and comfortable during your daily activities. For instance, if you are using absorbent pads, always keep a few in a plastic bag in your purse in case you need them. You may also want to keep other supplies on hand, such as wet wipes or odor control products. Having a change of clothes in your car may come in handy in an emergency.

In Conclusion

We hope that the information provided in this book has given you a better understanding of urinary incontinence and the many ways it can be treated. Our greatest hope is that in reading this book, you will discover that you do not need to suffer in silence from the involuntary loss of urine.

Although this book explains numerous types of treatments, it should not be considered a substitute for a consultation with a doctor. We encourage you to visit a qualified medical professional who can recommend a treatment plan for you. The chances are very good that with the right type of treatment, your incontinence may be controlled, and you may start enjoying your life more.

Resources

American Urogynecologic Society Foundation
2025 M Street Northwest, Suite 800
Washington, DC 20036
Phone: 202–367–1167
Fax: 202–367–2167
Email: info@augsfoundation.org
www.augs.org

The American Urogynecologic Society Foundation provides public education programs and research for the treatment and cure of urogynecologic disorders, including incontinence. The organization's Web site includes detailed diagnostic and treatment information for incontinence, and a voiding diary is available for download free of charge. In addition, a physician finder feature lets you locate a urogynecologist near you.

American Urological Association Foundation
1000 Corporate Boulevard
Linthicum, MD 21090
Phone: 1–866–RING–AUA (746–4282) or 410–689–3700
Email: aua@auanet.org
www.urologyhealth.org

The American Urological Association Foundation was created to improve the prevention, detection, treatment, and cure of urologic disease. To achieve this goal, the foundation supports and promotes research, patient/public education, and advocacy. The organization's patient education Web site is written and reviewed by urology experts and provides information about urologic conditions, such as bladder control problems. The site also features a physician finder where you can search for a urologist in your area.

Interstitial Cystitis Association (ICA)
110 North Washington Street, Suite 340
Rockville, MD 20850
Phone: 1–800–HELP–ICA (435–7422) or 301–610–5300
Fax: 301–610–5308
Email: icamail@ichelp.org
www.ichelp.org

Established in 1984, the ICA offers support and information to IC patients and their families, educates the medical community about IC, and promotes research for the treatment of IC and, ultimately, to find a cure for IC. The ICA's Web site offers a monthly news digest, information on clinical trials and experimental therapies, answers to patient questions, and local and national patient support.

National Association for Continence (NAFC)
P.O. Box 8306
Spartanburg, SC 29305-8306
Phone: 1–800–BLADDER (1–800–252–3337)
www.nafc.org

Dedicated to improving the quality of life of people with incontinence, this nonprofit organization is a leading source for education and advocacy. The NAFC offers consumer-friendly information on the causes, prevention, diagnosis, and treatment of incontinence as well as on managing incontinence. The organization's numerous resources include a quarterly newsletter, a support group kit, and a comprehensive index to incontinence products and services.

National Institute of Diabetes and Digestive and Kidney Diseases (NIDDK)
National Kidney and Urologic Diseases Information Clearinghouse (NKUDIC)
3 Information Way
Bethesda, MD 20892-3580
Phone: 301–654–4415
http://kidney.niddk.nih.gov

The NKUDIC distributes information for the National Institute of Diabetes and Digestive and Kidney Diseases
(NIDDK). The NIDDK is part of the National Institutes of
Health, which is part of the U.S. Department of Health and
Human Services. Established in 1987, the NKUDIC aims to
educate the general public and health-care professionals
about diseases of the kidneys and urologic system, including
incontinence. The NKUDIC offers a number of services and
resources geared to the general public, including responses
to inquiries about kidney and urologic diseases, free publi-
cations, and referrals to health-care professionals.

Simon Foundation for Continence
P.O. 835-F
Wilmette, IL 60091
Phone: 1–800–237–4666
www.simonfoundation.org

The Simon Foundation's mission is to: "bring the topic of incontinence out of the closet, remove the stigma surrounding
it, and provide help and hope to people with incontinence,
their families and the health professionals who provide their
care." The foundation's Web site offers educational materials, a database of incontinence products, and a section
where individuals with incontinence can share their stories
and experiences with others.

Glossary

Alpha-adrenergic inhibitors: Medications that relax the bladder neck and urethra.

Alpha-adrenergic stimulants: Medications that cause the bladder neck and urethra to tighten.

Anticholinergics: Medications that block nerve impulses to the bladder.

Atrophic urethritis: The wasting away of the tissues of the urethra.

Atrophic vaginitis: The wasting away of the tissues of the vagina.

Autologous tissue: Tissue that comes from your own body.

Catheter: A hollow tube inserted into the urethra to allow for drainage of urine.

Cholinergics: Medications that stimulate the nerves that send signals to the bladder.

Collagen: A protein found naturally in humans and animals.

Cystocele: Bladder prolapse.

Cystogram: A test that involves the use of X-rays to view the bladder as it fills and voids; also called a video urodynamics study.

Cystometry: A urodynamic test that measures bladder pressure.

Cystoscope: A long, slender tube with a camera on the tip that is used to visualize the bladder and urethra and used for the passage of surgical instruments into the bladder and urethra.

Cystoscopy: A diagnostic exam that allows a doctor to see inside the bladder and urethra.

Diuretics: Agents that increase urine production and excretion; also called water pills.

Enterocele: Small bowel prolapse.

Fascia: Connective tissue in the human body.

InterStim Therapy: A sacral nerve stimulator that is implanted surgically to treat overactive bladder and urge incontinence.

Interstitial cystitis: Chronic inflammation of the bladder wall.

Intrinsic sphincteric deficiency: A type of stress incontinence in which the urethral sphincter is unable to close tightly enough to prevent urine loss.

Kegel exercises: Exercises that strengthen the muscles of the pelvic floor.

Laparoscope: A long, thin rod with a camera at the tip that is inserted into small incisions during surgery.

Leak point pressure: The amount of bladder pressure that causes urinary leakage.

Minimally invasive midurethral sling: A surgical procedure involving small incisions for the insertion of a sling to provide support for the bladder and urethra.

Needle suspension: Bladder neck suspension procedure in which long needles are used to pass sutures through incisions.

Nocturia: Frequent urination at night.

Occlusive devices: Medical devices, such as urethral pads and inserts that block the urethra to prevent urine from escaping.

Pad test: A diagnostic test used to determine the amount of urinary leakage being experienced.

Pelvic organ prolapse: A pelvic organ that has dropped out of its normal anatomical position.

Persistent incontinence: Incontinence that is typically due to underlying physical problems.

Pessary: A medical device worn to support the pelvic organs.

Polyuria: Excessive urine output.

Postvoid residual test: A urodynamic test that measures the amount of urine remaining in the bladder after urination.

Pubovaginal sling procedure: A surgical procedure to treat stress incontinence using incisions in the vagina for the insertion of a sling to provide support for the bladder and urethra.

Rectocele: Rectum prolapse.

Retropubic suspension: A bladder neck suspension procedure using abdominal incisions.

Retropubic technique: A surgical technique used in sling procedures using abdominal incisions.

Suprapubic tube: A tube inserted into the bladder through an incision in the abdomen to allow for drainage of urine.

Transient incontinence: Temporary incontinence that is treatable.

Transobturator technique: A surgical technique used in sling procedures using incisions in the creases of the inner thigh.

Ureters: Two tubes that carry urine from the kidneys to the bladder.

Urethral hypermobility: A type of stress incontinence in which the urethra moves up and down rather than tightening when external pressures occur.

Urethral pressure profile: A urodynamic test that evaluates the urethra's ability to close.

Urethral sphincter: The muscle surrounding the urethra that closes it to prevent urine loss.

Urodynamic testing: A series of diagnostic tests used to evaluate bladder function.

Uroflowmetry: A urodynamic test that measures how fast urine is excreted.

Urogynecologist: A medical doctor who specializes in female urinary disorders.

Urologist: A medical doctor who specializes in the field of urology.

Urology: A field of medicine that focuses on the urinary and reproductive systems.

Video urodynamics study: A test that involves the use of X-rays to view the bladder as it fills and voids; also called a cystogram.

Voiding diary: A written record of fluid intake, urination, and episodes of leakage.

Voiding study: A urodynamic test that involves recording pressure changes in the bladder and urethra.

Index

About the Authors

"As a physician and surgeon, I thrive on the challenge of seemingly difficult problems. I respect the privilege of the trust my patients have given me, and I admire their endless strength "
—Michael H. Safir, M.D.

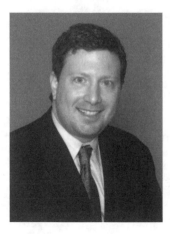

MICHAEL H. SAFIR, M.D., is a reconstructive urologist in Los Angeles and the San Fernando Valley. He currently serves as chairman of surgery at West Hills Hospital and is director of the Center for Reconstructive Surgery at Miracle Mile Medical Center.

Dr. Safir is a graduate of Northwestern University Medical School (Honors Program in Medical Education). He completed his residency in urology at the same institution. Following residency training, he completed fellowship training at the University of California, San Francisco and UCLA medical schools in the fields of reconstructive urology and female urology. Dr. Safir served as a clinical instructor at UCSF and UCLA medical schools and served as assistant professor and section chief of Reconstructive and Female Urology at New York Medical College.

Dr. Safir specializes in the treatment of urinary incontinence, repair of pelvic prolapse, and reconstructive genitourinary surgery. He is the coauthor of many textbook chapters, including a chapter in The Oxford Textbook of Surgery on urinary disorders. He lives in Los Angeles with his wife, Robyn, and two children.

Dr. Safir may be reached at his Web site www.drsafir.com or via e-mail at dr@drsafir.com.

"I became a urologist because the specialty uses both medical and surgical approaches in treating patients as individuals, with emphasis on maintaining their personal dignity. My post-graduate training, military experience, and clinical practice in the aftermath of Hurricane Katrina have only reinforced that philosophy."
— Clay N. Boyd, M.D.

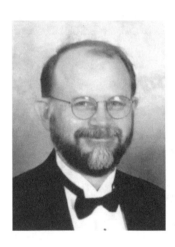

CLAY N. BOYD, M.D., is a board-certified urologist who has been in private practice in the River Parishes region of Greater New Orleans, Louisiana. He evaluates and treats urinary incontinence as part of his practice.

Dr. Boyd is a summa cum laude graduate of the University of Southern Louisiana (now the University of Louisiana at Lafayette) in Lafayette, Louisiana. He received his medical degree from Louisiana State University Medical Center, New Orleans, where he holds a position in the Department of Urology of LSU Health Sciences Center. He completed his surgical internship and residency in urology at Charity Hospital of New Orleans, followed by active duty service as urology section chief at the 92nd Strategic Hospital with the rank of major in the United States Air Force, departing with honorable discharge with commendation.

Dr. Boyd is a member of the American Urological Association, Orleans Parish and Louisiana State Medical Societies, and Louisiana Health Care Review. He is also an active member of the Air Force Association, as well as of the New Orleans World Trade Center. His enrollment for the HealthCare MBA program through George Washington University School of Business has been accepted.

Dr. Boyd may be reached at LSU Health Sciences Center Department of Urology at www.medschool.lsuhsc. Edu/urology_dept/.

*"Treating patients who suffer from urinary incontinence
is a very gratifying area of medicine to practice. The loss of
urinary control can be devastating and can greatly limit the
social aspects of patients' lives. Giving that control back
to people is very rewarding."*
— Tony E. Pinson, M.D.

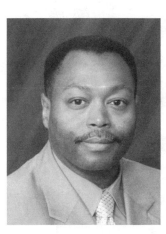

TONY E. PINSON, M.D., is a board-certified urologist who specializes in urinary incontinence and female urology. Dr. Pinson is a graduate of the University of Michigan School of Medicine. He completed his general surgery training at SUNY Upstate University in Syracuse, New York, and his urological training at the University of New Mexico in Albuquerque, New Mexico. He is currently owner of Pinson Urology and Continence Center, P.C., in the mid-Michigan area.

Dr. Pinson is a member of the American Urological Association and is a fellow of the American College of Surgeons. He is a frequent urological consultant and adviser for multiple multinational companies. He has served as chief of staff at W. A. Foote Memorial Health System and as medical director of the Jackson Outpatient Surgery Center. Dr. Pinson is very active in his community of Jackson, Michigan, where he serves on numerous community boards and maintains his private practice. He is married and has two sons.

More information can be obtained about Dr. Pinson at www.Pinsonurology.com.

Addicus Books Consumer Health Titles
Visit our online catalog at www.AddicusBooks.com

Organizations, associations, corporations, hospitals, and other groups may qualify for special discounts when ordering more than twenty-four copies. For more information, please contact the Special Sales Department at Addicus Books. Phone (402) 330-7493. Email: info@AddicusBooks.com

Book Order Form

Please send:

_____ copies of _____

at_____each.

Total_____

Nebraska residents add 6.5% sales tax _____

Shipping/Handling_____

$4.60 postage for first book:_____

$1.10 for each additional book: _____

TOTAL ENCLOSED _____

Name _____

Address_____

City _____State _____Zip_____

☐ Visa ☐ MasterCard ☐ American Express ☐ Discover

Credit card number_____

Expiration date _____

Ways to Order:

- Mail order by credit card, personal check, or money order. Send to: Addicus Books, P.O. Box 45327, Omaha, NE 68145

- Order TOLL FREE: 800-352-2873

- Online at www.AddicusBooks.com